OLDER AND BOLDER

OLDER AND BOLDER

HARRY PHILLIPS

NAVIGATOR

Published by Navigator Books
Ringwood, Hampshire, England.

Copyright © Harry Phillips

ISBN 0 902830 30 9

A CIP catalogue record for this book is
available from the British Library

Typeset by Moorhouse Typesetters
Printed by The Cromwell Press, Melksham, Wiltshire.

A book of recollections, facts,
stories and nostalgia, recalling
the times that pensioners have
lived through.
An attempt to explain why it
has come about that the ELDERLY
are not getting a very good deal
in old age.
A rallying call to fight for the
rights that we have earned in
service to our country.

EVERYONE OVER 55
SHOULD VOTE FOR
THE ELDER PARTY

There are 14,667,949 OVER 55s in the U.K., enough votes to form a Political Party of our own, the ELDER PARTY, (EP).
The problems of the 55 - 65 age group are discussed in Chapter Nine.

CHAPTER ONE

Meanwhile, from the pensioner's viewpoint, the Elderly are not having a very happy time, but could improve their lives considerably by voting for a Political Party of their own.

Once upon a time it seemed to us that retirement meant taking it easy, slippers and the armchair, peace, time for the grandchildren, pottering about the garden, roses round the door, basking in the respect accorded to old age.

Suddenly all this seems to be different, partly because this view of 'old' was our view when we were younger, and now we are there, now that we are old

1

ourselves the scene has been allowed to change.

Not that the old can be lumped together as a single group of Over 60/65s; every human variety imaginable inhabits the world of the old, but once you receive your pension you enter that world.

Specialists, (under Age 65 but who nevertheless know all about being Over 65), tell us that our time is now ours to spend as we choose, that we can expect to live in retirement nearly as many years as we did at work, that we must make good use of this time, discover new talents, study, attend classes, join clubs, play scrabble, chess or bridge, be a volunteer. We are not expected, apparently, to exercise an influence on the affairs of our country or on our destiny.

The gap between haves and have-nots amongst the elderly is increasing, with commercial entrepeneurs targeting the Third Age market; but although a comfortable number of pensioners have a comfortable life, the average pensioner in the U.K. is having a hard time and what makes it more difficult to bear is that our particular generation of old are the men and women who went to war, experienced danger and millions dying, to give this country and many other countries, the freedom that everybody takes for granted today. We were needed then, we had an influence on the destiny of our country then; and we can have an influence on the destiny of our country now if we stir ourselves to do something about it.

To previous generations of old we gave respect; now that our turn has come, what we receive, mainly, is neglect. We are constantly reminded that we are causing a problem for a Government which has got its finances into a mess by getting its priorities wrong. If you ask the Government why pensioners in other countries get bigger pensions than we do they avoid giving a reply by pontificating about their so called achievements.

Money is certainly the root of pensioners' problems, and until you have experienced a life of scratching for pennies you have no idea how such a permanent condition of anxiety can get you down, affecting your whole life. Scrabble, chess or bridge can't lift the hearts of the empty purse and pocket brigade. The money that the Post Office clerk pushes across the counter to you each week already has wings, allocated, gone, and items like joints of meat, even semi-luxury foods are a long forgotten dream this week, next week, for ever. Nothing is likely to change, except the possibility of your being mugged for your pension in broad daylight on your way home from collecting it. Nothing is likely to change unless we make the effort to change, and we have the voting numbers to do so.

It is now realised that, although in the majority of

cases today, the health of the elderly is reasonably good, the spirit is most definitely not. A newspaper article reports that there is a large, silent group of people in Britain today who feel under siege, cut off from their families and outside the mainstream of society; they are the generation who hoped for a better old age than society offers them today.

There is no doubt whatever that the elderly and the old are the most deserving section of the community. When they were young they had to suffer restrictions on a scale that the young of today could not begin to contemplate. Some of the older ladies began life in an age when women didn't even have a vote, and as for becoming pregnant before marriage, they would have had to endure nothing but disgrace. You can understand the bitterness felt by the old ladies at the benefits showered on unmarried mothers today, including accommodation better than their own. It is in their power to change it.

Most elderly, though not ill, have somehow been ground down to third class citizen level by an inconsiderate, cold, uncaring society; apart from anxiety bombshells like the poll tax and the tax on fuel, they have lost, and certainly do not have the basic quality of life to enable them to adopt a more optimistic attitude to living. Laughter, it is said, is decidedly life enhancing, but the majority of the elderly have little to laugh about these days. But they could have. For too long we have accepted that we are at the bottom of the heap, that because we are pensioners we are at the mercy of the smart 40-year old politicians. We must realise that we have the voting numbers to vote for ourselves, to decide our own futures and that of the country.

IF YOU ARE OLD AND RICH

If you are old and wealthy, and particularly if you are disgustingly rich, you will probably be giving some of it away for the sake of your immortal soul, aware that the Bible tells us to share what God has given us with those in need; but it is not enough just to instruct some fawning financier or servile solicitor to set up a trust which requires from you no more physical inconvenience than signing your name on a deed or cheque. You have got to engage in a little personal involvement.

Find out a few of the needy yourself and see that they get care, joints of meat, bags of coal, food parcels, bottles of Scotch, holidays, organise taking war widows to the graves of their husbands. Make an effort not to be pompous, do it humbly without expecting forelock tugging and genuflecting all over the place. Whatever you do, you must do it anonymously, but you must also be physically involved if you want the dear Lord to pat you on the head later on. You've got a lot more than most people to answer for when you turn up at the Pearly Gates, a lot of stewardship that you've been entrusted with, and you'd be wise to start earning some Immortal Bonus Points right away if you don't want to spend a few thousand years doing penance down a spiritual coal mine.

The Lord has already denied you a range of emotional thrills available to the rest of humanity because,

everything diminishes in value in relation to your ability to afford it

the greatest enjoyment in life is the realisation of things most often denied you

Another thing. There must be many political decisions made that affect your interests. A fraction of your wealth could help to create our own political party and then you might have a say in influencing decisions of benefit to you and the cause of the elderly generally.

BETWEEN THE POOR OLD AND
THE RICH OLD ARE MANY
IN BETWEEN OLD WITH GOOD
HEALTH AND ENOUGH MONEY
BUT NOT GETTING ENOUGH
OUT OF LIFE.
TO THEM I WOULD SAY

Make an effort not to talk old or think old or to walk old. Never, never whinge "I'm 75, you know, or 85 or whatever ..." so what?

Never talk about yourself unless asked, always take more interest in your companion.

If your years are your only excuse for sympathy you have no excuse to seek it until your age really shows.

If you act like a poor old so-and-so that's how the world will treat you.

Get your mind off feeling sorry for yourself and take an interest in something. Don't just sit there on your backside being old. There is a cause waiting for you to fight, a cause to excite you out of bed in the morning, a cause to get your adrenalin going at the prospect of power.

You might be a bit slower than you were, but so are people of 45. Your brain can be just as good,

8

your life can be full and contented, right to the end. Obviously you're not likely to be asked to run the hundred yards or climb Everest, in fact you're not likely to be asked to do anything that you are not capable of doing, so don't develop an automatic, "Oh, I couldn't do that" response. Develop a 'have a go' mentality.

Attitude! That's it. This is the attitude you **should** have.

You could really come alive by involving yourself with the new ELDER PARTY.

With little effort you would link up with others of similar interests, making new friends, attending parties and other social occasions to further the EP cause. You could suddenly find yourself with a much fuller life, with the added satisfaction that what you were doing was worthwhile, of benefit not only to you but to those less fortunate than yourself. It could be an exciting cause, too.

BUT FOR MOST OF THE ELDERLY
LIFE IS HARD

Following the publication of my book, "*FAMOUS WAYS TO GROW OLD*," I have researched widely amongst older folk and my conclusions emanate from the majority of elderly I meet.

These days, the eleven million elderly, one fifth of the population, feel increasingly isolated and ignored, probably because they are isolated and ignored. Society has lost interest in them unless they have money or influence, without which the elderly are consigned to a life of no consequence, outside the mainstream of life. Bureaucrats patronise them and nobody really cares for their special concerns and interests. Community Care for the elderly has failed; 85% of doctors say that the service has deteriorated. Medical services are failing because of bureaucratic interference and through no fault of the splendid doctors and nurses involved. Various organisations find jobs for themselves by looking after the old, employing younger staff to do so, though mostly kind, considerate and conscientious, unaware that nobody knows about being old until they are old themselves.

Nobody really knows about anything until they have personal experience of it, getting really involved themselves. Of course you agonise when someone near to you gets cancer, for instance, but what a billion per cent difference it makes when you get cancer yourself.

Like old age; nobody knows about being old until they are old themselves which is why the active old, of whom there are more than sufficient numbers in need of something to do, should be in charge of the affairs of the old. Smart 40-year olds, who seem to rule our lives, assume that pensioners are has-beens but when you reach that age you realise, perhaps to your surprise, that your brain is as keen, tough and responsive as it has ever been. How old was Winston Churchill when he conquered the Axis powers? The Over 65s are capable of more than you realise, as will be suggested later.

When you're old, you realise that although there are obviously several stages of Old, from the moment of receiving your pension the indifference of society begins to be felt, an exclusion here and there, and a malaise creeps over your life like an incoming tide over the sandcastle of your social importance. We can fight that and shall be better for doing so; we shall fulfil our lives by doing so.

A report for the Carnegie Society discovered that

11

retired people spend as much time watching television as they did working, but that older people rarely appear in programmes in relation to their numbers in society.

The elderly are the largest, yet least noticed section of the community, only receiving publicity when they are driven to protest at some particularly harsh piece of legislation.

"We can assure you that the elderly *in need* will be given help with their heating bills," says nice Mr. Major.

> *"Sit by the fireside with Sorrow*
> *You with the unpaid bill, Despair."*

The elderly are well aware that help for the needy in meeting extra heating bills involves an inquisition that offends the dignity of those who have had to sacrifice so much throughout their lives. In making this sacrifice, few realised that they would need to be interrogated in order to establish their right to survival in old age. Let us not put up with this sort of treatment any more.

The younger generations will never comprehend the extent of the sacrifice freely offered by the elderly men and women of today, without which they would not know their present freedom.

Some of the modern generation can't seem to grasp

that it wasn't professional Armed Forces that won the war, it was us, clerks and tradesmen, workers and gents, from civvies one day to the Battle of Britain, Alamein, the Battle of the Atlantic and many other theatres of war.

A brief reminder of one of the events of those days may be appropriate. Winston Churchill said,

"Before Alamein we never had a victory.
After Alamein we never had a defeat."

... the guns opened fire and then the XXXth and X11th Corps advanced, attacking on a front of four divisions. XXXth Corps attempted to cut two corridors through the German lines. Two Xth Corps Armoured Divisions followed behind them. By dawn, despite progress, the minefields had not been penetrated in depth and there was no prospect of a breakthrough. The South African, 4th Indian Division, the 7th and 44th Divisions of X111th Corps attacked. For days hard fighting continued. Then the 9th Australian Division struck northwards towards the sea, finally isolating four German battalions; the ceaseless, bitter fighting of the Australians swung the whole battle in our favour ...

13,500 men of our generation were lost in twelve days at Alamein.

Many of us have our memories, something to be proud of indeed.

Considering this sacrifice, it is beyond belief that we, the present Retired, amongst whom are a large proportion of Ex-Service men and women, proud saviours of our nation, should rate so low in social regard and in Government welfare priorities. It is also beyond belief that we, The Retired, should not realise that we represent one fifth of the population and that we *can* do something about improving our lot and our position in life. Think about it. Later in the book I will explain how we can be a force to be reckoned with. The war was a cause that brought us all together in a spirit of comradeship and brotherhood. But for us, and the few million dead comrades that society barely remembers for just 2 out of the 525,600 minutes available in every year, our country, and ten other EC countries could well be Nazi States, even today. We need a cause like that again, though obviously not a war. For us elderly there is such a cause waiting. A cause that can improve our lot in life, restore our self esteem.

We can get back into life. You'd be amazed what you can do at any age if you have the incentive.

CHAPTER TWO

If you're ill you're ill and there's nothing you can do about it except ask God to give you comfort in bearing it. But you can be ill at any age. Old and Ill go together to the extent that parts wear out, but it is a fact that older people are becoming increasingly fit and active, despite lacking hope and interest. But if you fail your M.O.T. on heart, say, it only means that there are some things you can't do. So concentrate on the things you CAN do. If you believe that you're more likely to be ill because you're old, you will be. If you believe that life is going to treat you badly, it probably will.

This was always true, of course, and pessimists are hardly likely to turn into optimists on reaching retirement age, indeed the reverse is more likely. But if you've got any fight left in you at 65, try not to lose it just because you're classified as old. Our life batteries are charged by the adrenalin of interest in our lives - remove all interest and the system runs down which is the case with far too many of us today. The interest of being able to determine our own future is there, waiting for you to make a move.

We should be suitably gratified to hear from the knowledgable Under 65s that we are a valued resource that should not be wasted. Despite this flattery we are nevertheless described, statistically as persons 'not economically active.' We could produce some surprises.

Throughout working life, retirement is looked forward to as a release from toil and worry, an escape to a sort of holiday freedom. It takes but weeks of retirement to realise that such dreams of retirement are an illusion, that one is let out from work not to the flowering beauty of freedom but to the dull nothing of a void. A cause awaits that could fill that void, that could give you far more than the interest of a lifetime of working.

A recent Gallup poll reveals that what is called the Feel Good Factor is at an all time low. Since these findings reflect the state of the nation as a whole, what chance do the retired stand in present circumstances, with barely enough resources for survival. It is easily within our power to improve this situation.

The 1980s saw the emergence of an awareness of the Third Age, a hopeful acknowledgement that retirement marked not the end, but only the end of a stage and that, from then, people were physically and mentally capable of development and were in need of it. Apart from this aspect, apart from drawing a shutter down on a lifetime accumulation of experience, it was at least more widely realised that skills should be passed on, giving a benefit to the giver as well as to the receiver. (I have shipwright friends, for instance, who with minimum tools could, from scratch, fashion a beautiful yacht in teak, yet whose skills lie on the scrapheap of our profit-is-all society, lost to future generations for ever. And how many more crafts are being lost in this way, unless something is done about it?) Who better than our generation to understand what should, and could, be done.

In a few areas a new/old enthusiasm is emerging but it is against the general pattern of behaviour expected of old people. Old people are treated as old, not because they are old but because they have lost a place in society's scale of values. They are thought of, if at all, as past their sell-by date in a profit obsessed world, in retreat even, as though their skills were exhausted, of no value rather than with a value only slightly diminished, consigned to the scrappy yard of life despite having a lot more mileage left in them.

The old are sometimes as much to blame for this as the world rejecting them. By accepting a losing situation we lose; by realising our voting power we change our attitude and, in doing so, increase our chance of success.

At the age of 65 the working life of most UK males comes to an end whether they like it or not. Although he may well be as fit and mentally active as he was at 45, his opportunities are limited. How this could change!

For married women, the majority, there is obviously no such thing as retirement in the sense that men retire; the major difference to their lives is that they suddenly have a man about the house objecting to the bloody vacuum cleaner, and interfering in long established household routines.

In any case, women are more often concerned with the effects of ageing than with retirement. Once adjusted to the lessening of attention that her charms once attracted, and having survived the mid-life anxieties and depressions, many women even have fuller and more self assured lives than before. They find that age, for them, has nothing to do with their birth certificates but with how they feel. Many women of over 65 are as happy as they have ever been, but only if they have an adequate life style. Money is the most important factor in later years, with it one can cope with many problems.

Oddly enough, statistics show that women are less healthy than men in later life, although they live

18

longer than men.

Women show greater willingness to take part in social activities than their menfolk, who usually display reluctance through self consciousness; but once in, enjoy the acceptance and activity.

There is no doubt that those who make the effort to stay physically and mentally active stay healthier longer.

Mortality statistics tell us that women live longer where other considerations are equal. A contributory factor is that women don't retire, since it is the act of retirement that can often start the ageing process. the transition from a work routine to nothing. The change in the woman's life is certainly considerable when she suddenly finds herself spending every waking moment with a man she'd have loved to have done this with fifty years before. Few women find it easy, and fewer still receive the occasional kiss or embrace to help through the new experience of living each twentyfour hours together. The need for emotional adjustment is as great as it was in the adolescent years but, of course, Grown Ups don't acknowledge that they need such guidance.

Don't depend on retirement; in the years before, set up a little secret something, helpful from a money point of view, but mainly to keep the brain active, to retain a little hold and respect in the busy world that will otherwise reject you.

The later chapters of this book will open your mind to the possibility of a new, exciting interest. Don't accept retirement in the sense of believing that you have no influence in the world. You know that your brain is as good as it was at 45. Your experience is twenty years better. Believe that you have a role to play and a role will emerge.

CHAPTER THREE

Considering her age she moved quickly to the car, fastened her seat belt, fussed around in the mysterious way women do before they can seem to get a car moving, reached to turn the ignition key, and it wasn't there.

She banged on the steering wheel in frustration, then sounded the horn, looked impatiently towards the front door, then sounded the horn again.

Presently it opened and her husband looked out.

"Car keys," she shouted through the opened window, "car keys."

Pausing briefly, he nodded his understanding and disappeared, The keys would be on the hook in the kitchen. Even at his speed of movement it wouldn't take a second. Perhaps they weren't there? Who had used the car last?

The door opened and he came out to the car. She reached out through the window.

"Here you are, love," he said.

"What's this?"

*"A handkerchief.	You said you wanted a handkerchief."*

Despite her exasperation she couldn't help smiling as she pointed to the ignition and he understood. He lent in to the car and put his arm round her.

"Sorry, love."

Some women are not so sympathetic, and many more older men are hard of hearing than care to admit it. Too many wives get impatient with husbands who cannot hear; if he fails to understand she assumes that he is going soft in the head but he would understand if he could hear.

Failure to hear excludes him. If his contributions to conversations are met with, "we've already said that," he is reluctant to try again.

The odd thing is that the majority of such afflicted males insist that their hearing is perfectly alright, thankyou, and some perverse conceit prevents them from even considering the use of a hearing aid. If wives would insist, however, many a deteriorating relationship could be improved.

Hearing loss, particularly in men, is a contributory factor in ageing. So gradual is this deterioration in hearing efficiency that it creeps up almost unobserved, its effect not noticed. Male vanity plays a part, too, in not wanting to acknowledge a weakness of this nature, and certainly not to the extent of having their hearing tested and of needing a hearing aid. The wearing of a hearing aid condemns you as old whereas all men like to think of themselves as youthful and virile until FORCED to admit that they are not. If, say, a leg shortened at the same rate as hearing deteriorated, there would be many men going around with one leg twelve inches shorter than the other but claiming that they were not lame.

Male hearing loss is noticed by wives before being acknowledged by husbands. It is sad, but almost inevitable, that wives are irritated when their remarks are misinterpreted, or not heard. Hearing howlers cause family amusement that a man is supposed to laugh at when he is far from amused. A stage is reached when "it's no good telling him, he won't hear" when a special effort to speak up, for his sake, would help him enormously and keep him in the fold.

Women's conversation is not easy to follow at the best of times, with unconnected words and ideas fluttering in all directions like butterflies. Part of the unfathomable delight of women is that they seem to talk most when they have least to say. When a man's hearing is sharp he can pick up female speech as recorded, however diverse. When his hearing fails he endeavours to follow conversations through key words. If he is discussing politics or the economic situation with a male companion it is likely that they will go on discussing politics and the economic situation, with key subject words recognisable, almost anticipated.

With his wife, or many woman, she will tell him that the vacuum cleaner has gone wrong, for instance, but as his hearing mechanism understands and zeros in on the subject of vacuum cleaners she is talking about the price of baked beans at Safeway, and by the time he gets that on his hearing wavelength she is wittering on about the 3-piece suite that her sister's son's girlfriend has bought, or some other inconsequential rubbish.

Failure to follow the discussion of two women should not be put down to hearing loss since they invariably both talk together at any age, climbing over each other's conversation without the slightest embarrassment or, presumably, understanding. This is one reason why women usually get their facts wrong but you should not put it down to your lack of hearing that you are unable to understand them.

Wives never seem to understand the need to speak up, to take the trouble to speak more clearly to a hard of hearing husband. They go on talking exactly as they have all through married life, aware of relationships getting scratchier, and not realising that if they would make an effort to speak clearly, their lives together could be happier. In any case, they shout in repeating what they have said so why not make themselves understood the first time.

People who can hear are invariably indifferent to the problems of those who can't, and that goes for relatives, too; indeed, hearing deficiency is often a cause of annoyance and hostility in families.

If someone would invent a recording machine that could play back to a wife exactly how much of her conversation her husband had been able to hear, she would probably find that less than half of her words were getting through.

Hearing people sometimes wonder why you don't say you can't hear; but hard of hearing people don't like to admit it. A large number of two way conversations are carried on with one party struggling to hear. Some voices are easier to pick up than others. (Salesmen and women should check on their performance in this respect; if the guy can't hear you he isn't likely to buy. Also, do public speakers who preface their speech with "Can you hear me there in the back?" expect someone to get up and reply "I can't hear you asking me if I can hear you."). If you start a conversation with someone who speaks quietly it would be better to admit that you can't hear them unless they speak up; at least this is a sensible prelude to a conversation that has a purpose, or at the beginning of a car journey, for instance, since conversations in cars have to compete with road noises.

But a great deal of verbal to-ing and fro-ing goes on in the normal day. and it gets tiresome to have to explain to the butcher, baker and candlestick maker that you can't hear.

Perhaps it would be a good idea for hard of hearing folk to be distinguished in some way, by a mark on the forehead like a caste mark, for instance. This would be the signal for people to be aware of their impairment in the hope that they might speak up.

A good idea? The obvious snag is that hard of hearing folk don't want to be regarded as such, and are acutely self-conscious when it is even suggested that they can't hear. So much so, that one of the big selling points of the Hearing Aid Manufacturers is that their aids are inconspicuous, the assumption being that if they did not pander to the conceit of their customers they would not have so many.

It is odd that a hearing aid should be detrimental to the manly image whereas glasses are universally worn without comment.

"Did you notice he had a hearing aid?"

The National Health hearing aid is as effective as private aids. The NH aid is free and private aids can cost up to a thousand pounds and more. The NH aid is visible and the private aid is not. Private aids sell very well.

Hearing aids are useful in situations where there is no distracting sound. Wearing hearing aids in crowded rooms you can but lipread your companion against a clashing patchwork of sound

Finally, a husband and wife relationship can be considerably improved if you will openly discuss hearing problems and do something about them.

ANOTHER SUGGESTION TO IMPROVE THE QUALITY OF YOUR LATER LIFE

"But we couldn't move," he said, "not with all the junk we've accumulated here."

"It would be nice, though," his wife replied. "Somewhere smaller, even a bungalow or a flat. Not to have so much work to do."

Later, she went up to the box room and looked around at the muddle; an old pram, a tennis racket, vases, boxes of clothes and papers. What was the point of keeping it all? One cardboard box, not standing level, was spilling its contents, a green and gold photo album attracted her.

Sepia prints brought back to her their smiling daughter; smiling then before the quarrel that had split the family.

"Never," her husband had raged, "never do I wish to have anything to do with her again."

Standing there in the dusty room it suddenly came to her what a stupid word 'never' was. And so, in the days that followed, when her husband was out, she made enquiries.

One evening, after dinner, when he was sitting in his armchair, she telephoned a number from the extension telephone in the kitchen.

"Phone," she called to him and he picked up the telephone by his armchair. She listened for a moment, almost overcome with emotion, then quietly put down the receiver and stood still, cold with fear. What would he say to her for doing that? It could even make him ill, he had felt so strongly about it. But ten minutes later, when she quietly lifted the receiver in the kitchen, they were still talking. She went in to her husband and saw that tears were streaming down his face. He held out his arm to her, to embrace her.

"Come here, talk to her ... she's coming ... we're going to be together again ..."

Is there someone in your life you have vowed never to speak to again? Is there someone with whom a quarrel stands, a secret cancer of bitterness within you, poisoning you?

Forgiveness is the most beautiful emotion, particularly if you are old you MUST forgive. If you have someone to forgive, you are lucky. There is no surer way of lifting up your heart, of bringing forgotten sunshine into your life, and, quite probably, into the lives of members of your family who would also benefit emotionally by your forgiveness.

Do it now. Pick up the telephone, write a letter. No conditions, forgive absolutely.

WHATEVER YOU MAY THINK ABOUT IT, HAVING FAITH IS A COMFORT AS YOU GET OLDER

Tiptoeing into the bedroom he saw that his wife was still asleep, and he carefully cleared a space on her bedside table to put down the breakfast tray. The red rose had fallen on to the toast and he moved it so that it showed to advantage against the white tray cloth.

Normally his entry with the tea tray woke her immediately, but after her accident yesterday, the doctor was coming again this morning to find out whether any serious implications were likely.

Should he wake her before the tea was cold? Instead, he knelt, rested his hands very lightly on the bedclothes covering her, closed his eyes and prayed that she would be alright.

Turning to her, as he prepared to get up, he was surprised to find that her eyes were wide open, matching a quizzical expression on her face.

"I didn't know you prayed," she said.

"How are you?"

"I'm alright, but I didn't know you prayed, after all these years, fancy. I pray, too, but I didn't think you'd

... I didn't like to ..."
They held hands and prayed together and a special
peace came over him.

Do you pray together? Or would you feel self
conscious at suggesting it? It's worth a little effort to
make a start; if it works, the jagged bits of life get
smoother, particularly comforting in later years.
There is a power there waiting for you to try together.
As Viscount Tonypandy said, "It must be terrible to
be old and not to believe in God's purpose."

CHAPTER FOUR

The age pyramid of the European Community shows a shrinking base as the result of a falling birthrate, and an expanding apex because the population is living longer. The two oldest regions in the community are Germany and Italy, in that they were the only two countries where fewer than 23% of the population are under 20.

Four years ago the median age of the Community population was 34.3 years compared with the age of the population of the world, estimated to be 24. The Federal Republic of Germany at 37.2 and Denmark at 35.6 were the oldest.

A quarter of the total Community population was under 20, and one fifth was over 60. With the population growing older, it is forecast that the proportion of young people to old will be equal by the year 2010, after which old people will be in the

32

majority from 2020 onwards.

In the northern EU countries, pensions are the largest single item of welfare state spending.

Germany (West)	47%
Italy	47%
France	42%
U.K.	34%

The percentage of GDP taken up by pensions, (1988 latest figures):-

Italy	10.7%
France	9.7%
U.K.	8.4%
Ireland	4.9%

Spain, Ireland, Greece and Portugal spend less than half the EU average.

Recent Eurostat figures show that how much of the GDP is taken up by Social Protection varies from 17% in Portugal to 30.7% in the Netherlands. The largest share of social benefits is devoted to old age at 45%, followed by Health at 36%.

Belgium, Denmark, France, Germany and Luxembourg all devoted more of their GDP to Social Benefits, (27% to 29%), than the U.K., Italy and Ireland where it was 23%, but better than Spain and Portugal at 17%.

Money paid out in benefits has obviously got to come from somewhere and there are three sources, contributions paid by the pensioner, by employers and by the Government.

The highest contribution from public funds is in Denmark at 78%, the lowest Netherlands at 14%, with the U.K. in the middle at 43.4%.

Employers' contributions were highest in Italy at 53% and lowest in Denmark at 4%, the U.K. figure being 27.9%.

Pensioners contributions were highest in Italy at 53% and lowest in Denmark at 4%, the U.K., 17%.

In Catholic Italy, Spain and Portugal, where unmarried motherhood carries a social stigma, there is no state provision.

But Denmark and Holland provide 60% of the average national income, Belgium 59%, France 50%, Luxembourg 35%, Greece 32%.

Using Eurostat 1990 comparitive figures, the Single Pension in the U.K. is shown as £54 per week. In the Netherlands it is £69 per week and in Denmark £79. It obviously varies from country to country, as does the cost of living. In a comparitive list of 68 countries where the most expensive country to live in, (Libya), appears as Number 1, Britain appears in 56th place.

A comparision of Means Tested Benefits for those without other resources is of interest.

(Source: Social Protection in the Member States of the Community 1991)

Netherlands	367
Italy	331
Belgium	322
Denmark	261
France	227
Ireland	206
Spain	172
U.K.	172
Germany	165
Italy	142

In the last thirty years the number of Over 60s in the EU has risen from 46.5 to 68.6 million, an increase of almost 50%. As already mentioned, it is estimated that this trend will continue and that in 2020 there will be approximately twice as many elderly in the EU as there were in 1960. Life expectancy assumptions predict 89 to 100 million elderly in the EU in 2020 of whom 17 to 22 million will be over 80.

In the whole of the EU, the elderly average 19.9% of the population. Figures for each country are:

Belgium	20.7%
U.K.	20.7%
Italy	20.6%
Germany	20.4%

Denmark	20.3%
Greece	20.2%
France	19.3%
Luxembourg	19.1%
Spain	18.95
Portugal	18.2%
Netherlands	17.4%
Ireland	15.3%

95% of the elderly live in private houses. Figures for the remainder living in nursing homes are not available.

In Germany, France and Greece there are legal obligations to provide care for their elderly. In Italy, Spain and Portugal the family is the focus of a tradition of collective responsibility which they must provide because of the lack of formal services.

The percentage of 80-year olds living on their own is highest in the Netherlands, nearly 60%, then Germany, the U.K., 55%, Belgium and France, below 50%, Italy and Luxembourg, about 40%, Ireland 35%, Greece, 28% and Spain, 17%. In the U.K. the elderly should be thankful that, unlike some other European elderly, we have not seen our family roots destroyed by war and ethnic hatred; for many, the map of Europe and, indeed, the world has been re-drawn in our lifetime, with consequent upheaval and distress.

Amongst European countries, more old people survive in Sweden (18.5% over 65 and 8.3% over 75), than in any other country. The smallest percentage of elderly survival is in Romania, (9.5% and 3.7%), and what was Yugoslavia, (1988 figures 9.1% and 3.8%). The U.K. comes in between with 15.6% and 6.9%.

The retirement age in other EU countries is: Male and Female

Italy	60 .. 55
Belgium	60 .. 60
France	60 .. 60
Greece	65 .. 60
U.K.	65 .. 60
Portugal	65 .. 62
Germany	65 .. 65
Spain	65 .. 65
Ireland	65 .. 65
Luxembourg	65 .. 65
Netherlands	65 .. 65
Denmark	67 .. 67

(there are provisions for variations)
(The U.K. female pension age will rise to 65 in 2020).

One would imagine that the skills and experience of older folk would be in demand by employers in the EU but this is not the case. There are 4.3 million men and 2 million women over age 60 working in the EU, or 10% of the total in this age group, almost one quarter of whom work in agriculture.

As in the U.K., there are many competent and

experienced Over 60s at the mercy of incompetent and inexperienced 40-year old politicians; as in the U.K. they could use their voting power to advantage.

The biggest problem for all European countries is the growing number of elderly folk in their populations.

Almost half of all elderly are between 60 and 69.
Almost one third are between 70 and 79.
The remaining 17.4%, 11.9 million, are over 80.

Not only are the total numbers of the elderly rising but the old are becoming older. About 10% of elderly were over 80 in 1960, today the figure is almost 17%. The forecast for 2020 is between 19 and 22% of elderly to be over 80. (In the year 2000 there is a temporary decline because of the decline of births in WW1).

In the 60 to 64 age group there are roughly the same number of men as women. In the 80 to 84 group there are two women to every man, and in the 90 to 94 group there are three women to every man.

The majority of women over 75 are widows.

Wars not only affect the number of deaths but the number of children being born; thus, in war time, male deaths are high, births low and the effect on the pensions requirement sixtyfive years later is apparent.

In World War One three quarters of a million men from Britain were killed, plus 200,000 from the Commonwealth.

In the Second World War a total of thirtyfive million, from all countries, were killed.

As a century which has seen two world wars draws to its close, there are obviously more old ladies than old gentlemen. There are almost two elderly ladies to each elderly man in Germany, for instance, at the other extreme, in Greece the proportion is eight men to ten women.

Whatever EU country you examine you find that female life expectancy is greater than male, although the extent of this difference varies. In France, sex difference in life expectancy at birth is most noticeable, due perhaps to the drinking habits of the French male.

There are more elderly widows than widowers, not only because of war casualties but because women usually marry men older than themselves; and how many widows there are obviously depends on how many have ever married. In Bulgaria only 1% of elderly men have never married but in Ireland 25% of elderly men have never married.

In Ireland 42% of elderly women are widows; in Hungary 61%. There are most widows in Germany and fewest in Portugal.

Are we doing well out of belonging to the EU?
Didn't Mrs. T handbag the other countries in to giving Britain a massive allowance of ECUs? Didn't she get Britain's contributions into line so that we got more out of the Common Market than we paid in? It may not be so bad buying coal from Germany, (who produce it at three times the world price), thereby putting our miners on the scrapheap, and buying milk from France so that our farmers have to pour theirs down the drain, **if** we are benefitting overall by our membership of the EU.

WHO GETS MORE OUT OF THE EU THAN THEY PUT IN?

Greece gets	3.9% more
Spain gets	2.9% more
Ireland gets	2.4% more
Belgium gets	1.6% more
Portugal gets	1.1% more
Luxembourg gets	0.7% more
Italy gets	0.7% more
Denmark gets	0.5% more

WHO PUTS MORE INTO THE EU THAN THEY GET OUT?

Netherlands pays out   0.1% more than she receives
France pays out   1.5% more than she receives
U.K. pays out   3.0% more than we receive
Germany pays out   9.0% more than she receives

Obviously every country wants to get more out of the EU than they put in, creating a larger market is an ideal but not at any price. As matters stand, the EU logo of a circle of stars could well stand for a snowball of escalating cost. Imagine the cost of offices, secretaries, clerks, computers, cars, lunches, stationery, hotels, travel.

How do all the different countries speak to each other, for instance? Through interpreters, of course, 750 of them at a cost of £50 million a year. There are another 1,000 translating documents from Spanish to Greek and Finnish to French and so on.

It appears that the European Parliament costs £476 million a year to run, equal to £919,000 per Euro Member of Parliament.

Even those 26 MEPs who lost their seats in the recent Euro elections were paid £2.2 million compensation.

How many Euromembers does each country have?

Numbers of members and population

France has 87	....	56,614,000
Germany has 99	....	80,372,000
Italy has 87	....	57,193,708
U.K. has 87	....	56,467,000
Spain has 64	....	38,872,268
Netherlands has 31	....	15,240,000
Belgium has 25	....	9,928.000
Greece has 25	....	10,256,464
Portugal has 25	....	10,582.000
Denmark has 16	....	5,146,469
Ireland has 15	....	3,525,719
Luxembourg has 6	....	309,800

And how keen are the populations of each country to vote. At the last, (1994) Euro election the percentage of votes cast was:

Belgium	90.7%
Luxembourg	87.4%
Italy	81.5%
Greece	79.9%
Ireland	68.3%
Germany	62.4%
Spain	54.8%
Portugal	51.1%
France	48.7%
Holland	47.2%
Denmark	46.1%
U.K.	36.2%

Is our lack of enthusiasm due to lack of information, or lack of a Referendum opportunity perhaps.

What do we really pay to the EU? What do we get out of it?

Latest trade figures are somewhat bewildering to the uninitiated in that they show our trade with the rest of the world to be greater than our trade with the Common Market!

Despite this, we are told that the commercial opportunities of the Common Market are huge, in which case it would be reassuring to feel that instead of politicians and civil servants in charge we had some competent business brains looking after our interests.

(The EC Court of Auditors revealed in November 1993 that the cost to the EC of bad financial management and fraud amounted to ninety million pounds)

If we knew the true cost of belonging to the Common Market it would probably make our hair stand on end, but we must hope that the final result will be worth while.

CHAPTER FIVE

"Do not go gentle into that good night
Old age should burn and rave at close of day
Rage, rage against the dying of the light"
Dylan Thomas

The elderly may not rage, but they are universally and understandably upset at the dying of the principles and moral values that shaped their lives. It is bad enough to be deprived of physical comforts through failure to apply principles, but the spread of morally offensive behaviour is bound to contribute to the general unhappiness of society and to the elderly in particular.

With the monogamous two-parent family ceasing to be a dominant model in private life, values and morals are sliding away to an 'anything goes' society.

What principles this Government has, it appears to discover for itself solely through expediency and financial considerations. For example, an unmarried 17-year old girl has a baby and is not criticised, nor given the hard time society would have given her fifty years ago. She is given £65 a week and a bright council home, a much brighter home than many elderly have to endure. But in some countries, where principles matter, she would have been condemned and given nothing by her Government.

In view of our tolerant and generous, (and foolish?), treatment of girls who become unmarried mothers, the number naturally grew until it exceeded 50,000, causing an unsustainable strain on the national economy. Only then, with this and other disturbing influences creating financial problems, is the Government forced to seek some principle and announces what it chooses to call a Back to Basics campaign. The countries who condemned sex outside marriage from the outset didn't need to invent Back to Basics to cure financial ills. They didn't have such a problem because, as a country, they had principles.

Live births outside marriage in Italy and Greece barely doubled in the thirty years from 1960. In the U.K. they increased fivefold.

In the last ten years the pregnancy rate amongst Under-16s in Britain has increased by 27%, the highest in Europe.

Needless to say, the Health Secretary announces that something will be done to curb the number of under age pregnancies in the hope of halving the number by the turn of the century. The fact that it has been allowed to happen is a sad reflection on our Government and society. One can only feel sorry for schoolgirls whose pattern of life is demolished by such foolishness.

In contrast to the number of births to young mothers, the average age at childbirth within marriage rose to 27.8 years, the highest ever recorded.

Apart from unmarried mothers, if sufficient influential voices had condemned a permissive society we would undoubtedly have had fewer marital problems. The media obsession with sex and nightly doses of extra marital sex on our television screens would not have been there to loosen morals and infiltrate temptation.

In the 1950s there were less than 40,000 divorces granted annually to a population of over ten million women. In 1991 there were 168,249 in the U.K. We are surely still the same sort of people, but subject to different influences.

The 1991 Census showed 793,000 live births of which 236,000 were outside marriage. There were 165,500 legal abortions.

Most older people have stayed married. The younger generation seem to live together only so long as their partners remain wholly desirable and agreeable in every respect, children regardless.

And even those couples who do stay together, forming a two-parent family with the husband working and the wife caring for the children, are discriminated against, socially, morally and financially.

Many elderly folk are saddened to have at least one member of their family in a single parent state, a grandchild or great grandchild being brought up without the benefit of both natural parents.

It was the custom for old time relationships to accept their partner's imperfections, whereas today the answer is to try someone else, and then someone else in the futile expectation that the person of ones early acquaintance will stay that way. Relationships seem to have acquired different values since our day. Modern couples are not giving themselves a chance to fulful their natural roles as family and parents. Older people observe that the new sexual freedom does not appear to have brought greater happiness.

Britain has the highest percentage of one parent families in Europe. If the 20-year olds and 30-year olds think they are having a hard time today, they should give a thought to what their lonely life might be in forty or fifty years time. They should make an effort to understand that over the years and over the world, the majority of women who have persevered, have found the role of wife and mother to be fulfilling and wholly satisfying.

What causes amused boredom amongst the younger generation is when we older folk start sounding off about "when I was your age etc." Because we didn't have sex on early aquaintance when we were their age we are regarded as fuddy-duddies; maybe if such sexual freedom had been available in our young days we would have behaved in the same way, but it wasn't; the pity is that in our later financial years we are being made to bear the financial consequences of such sexual freedom, or carelessness, or stupidity today; for it is obvious that if money wasn't paid to unmarried mothers it would mean more available for pensioners.

When today's grandmothers were young, an 11-o-clock curfew was rigidly enforced by parents and this enforced rationing of sexual freedom prevented many of the problems experienced today. When we were young, if a girl 'got into trouble', the consequences for her and her bastard child were so degrading, wretched and uncomfortable that few girls took the risk. That sex wasn't readily available showed men up in an honourable light, but there was more to it than that, there was a loyalty that does not seem to exist today. Getting to know a partner had to rely on values other than sex so that, if the relationship continued it was based on those values and was more likely to endure.

In those days there was a greater religious

awareness too   The Government might not have been forced by monetary pressures to sermonise about returning to the social and moral values of years ago, if the Church had retained the influence to do so. Weakening of moral standards were brought about by apathetic majorities and active minorities; any sort of discipline being opposed, parents and schools denied the corrective punishments that had secured obedience amongst earlier generations

What an outcry there would have been if, at the beginning of the Unmarried Mother snowball the Church and the Government had had the guts to condemn it, and if child benefits had been refused in such circumstances in the expectation that by doing so they would stop the snowball rolling. Vociferous minority groups of twits and do-gooders would have been suitably outraged to defend the rights of girls to have babies if they wanted to, without a thought for the fact that, already, one in five children is brought up in poverty. Child benefit only goes a small way to meeting the cost of children, and there is no doubt whatever that single parent children are disadvantaged and will remain so. With a recent report claiming that child benefit needs to be increased, and the Government seeking to reduce the vast Child Benefit budget, a Government that had possessed the foresight and the guts to have taken a moral stand would have benefited the community it is supposed to serve.

If sufficient influential voices had condemned sex before marriage the State might not be paying millions, or is it now billions, to unmarried mothers today, nor providing them with bright homes when many elderly live in damp and cold. Even half of that money would change the lives of pensioners in need.

In promoting its 'Back to Basics' campaign, only now is the Government trying to recapture the qualities of life that we pensioners knew. If the promotion of 'Back to Basics' is a recognition that a national malaise exists, a malaise that deflates the quality of life of everybody in the country, what hope is there for the deserving elderly who come last in the consideration stakes, and will continue to come last, whatever party is in power, until they realise that they have the influence to do something about it.

Even without allowing for Government incompetence and waste, there is growing concern that if the State carries on in its present fashion it will be unable to support the enormous pensions bill for an ageing population in the first quarter of the next century. 50/55-year olds today should be concerned to take action today as suggested in later chapters.

An elderly gentleman said, "The pompous way the Government talk about the mess the country is in and how they will get us out of it; but who got us into it in the first place. You can't help the elderly numbers growing to be a greater strain on the community, but you could have forseen what was happening, and safeguarded the means to provide for them."

The present breed of politicians are continually overtaken by events in this way, lacking the intelligence or perception to see and plan ahead.

One in four children will not be spending Christmas with both their natural parents according to a recent report, and by the year 2000, it is predicted, only half of the nation's children will have the benefit of being brought up by their natural parents.

1994 has been designated by the United Nations as the International Year of the Family, and a recent survey finds that the key to a happy life is a happy marriage, and that a happy marriage elevates the quality of life of each partner. Persevering in the married relationship can obviously pay dividends for each partner.

If they would listen, we elder folk could say to foolish 20 to 30-year olds who reject a partner at a whim; when, at the age of 80, you can look across the candlelit table at your companion of how many years, your companion through angry exchanges and walkouts, loving and conflict, to look across the table with the glowing feeling that "I love you" - you really know in your soul that love is not bought cheaply, that true love is a sacrifice of part of each of you over years of test and trial.

let the punishment fit the crime

Most of us elderly were chastised with a cane when we were young and it didn't appear to do us any harm, indeed we fully realised what the punishment would be if we did wrong and behaved accordingly.

Newspaper publicity records the case of a 17-year old persistent offender who was sent on a £7,000 safari holiday. The trip was organised by a Special School in North Wales where the boy had been sent at a cost of £1,800 a week by the Gloucestershire Social Services Department; it was also used by other county social services. The Home Secretary and the Prime Minister duly condemned the extravagance, but why allow it in the first place? On such occasions, all too frequent, the Government are clearly irritated to have to admit that they don't know how the taxpayers' money is being spent.

Another teenage offender from the same £1,800 a week school was sent on a 80-day character building trip to Egypt and Kenya. He attacked a pensioner with a hammer and, despite his so-called character building has also been charged with drunk driving and possession of an offensive weapon. The pensioner involved said, "They should bring back the birch for people like him."

To keep an old person in a Government Approved Home, the Government thinks that a maximum of £191 a week is enough. To keep a young offender in a home suitable for them the Government thinks that £1,800 is suitable, not only suitable but a bargain since suitable Government homes for young offenders apparently cost more than this. Even with the absurdly expensive treatment, or more probably because of it, ALMOST THREE QUARTERS of young offenders re-offend.

Old people recall that, in their day, young offenders were punished with six strokes of the birch and it would be interesting to compare the juvenile delinquency figures of those days with the figures now. As late as 1920 the British Government legalised the use of the cat-o-nine-tails for those convicted of robbery but its use was confined to those convicted of assault, robbery and rape.

Many elderly, having received canings themselves when they were young, without harmful effects, deplore the present do-gooder attitude to criminals today, even to vicious thugs, rapists and murderers. Most elderly believe that for those who leave their victims beaten up, bloodied, raped and probably maimed for life, no punishment is too bad, and that these thugs, cowards that they are, could well be deterred at the prospect of corporal punishment.

When you see photographs of old ladies who have been brutally beaten by some strong, savage thug, utterly defenceless frail, gentle old ladies scarred and bloodied, how can anyone argue against flogging as the most suitable punishment for the evil perpetrators. Although they cause their victims to suffer, often for life, there is an immediate outcry from the do-gooders at any suggestion of physically punishing the criminals.

Meanwhile, recorded offences in England and Wales have risen from 3 million in 1981 to 5.6 million in 1992. Drug offences increased from 17,921 to 48,927.

Apparently, a number of juvenile delinquents are under the influence of drugs when they commit their crimes. Perhaps drugs are one of the biggest cause of the increase of crime during our lifetimes. The horrific injuries caused by drug crazed attackers is bad enough, but the saddest result of drug pushing activities is the death of young people hooked on heroin. Reading the report of a pretty 21-year old girl killed by this drug, how can one fail to be moved by the mother's words, "she got caught up in this web, and once they're in it, it's dreadful. We gave her all the love we could give, a comfortable home. I had to

54

watch my daughter die because of these evil pushers."

Unmarried mothers started at one and rose to over fifty thousand before the Government was stirred, (and then by financial and not moral pressure), to do something about it. Do the deaths of young people from heroin have to reach fifty thousand before the Government take tough measures?

In countries where penalties are physically tough there are fewer crimes.

If the law was amended so that anybody convicted of pushing drugs to young people received ten strokes of the birch rod it might save untold damage to young lives. There would be no shortage of angry parents to wield the cat-o-nine-tails, to punish the scum who ruin the lives of their children.

We seem to live in a world in which children of 17 or 18 are provided by a soft-headed Government with benefits, and even accommodation, to live on their own, simply because they say they can't get on with their parents; and the Government accommodates them.

The elderly can look back to times when 17 and 18-year respected their parents, (and their grandparents), and did what they were told, crime was low, when they could go out at night, even in the dark, society was orderly, homosexuals went to prison, and the great majority of men and women got married and stayed married. It is unhappy for the elderly to be so much affected by social and financial problems created by the collapse of these disciplines, disciplines that shaped our lives.

The Government will never develop the character to make real progress while their gutless attitude of wanting to be all things to all men persists. Afraid to offend unmarried mothers, ethnic minorities, sexual discrimination cranks, gays and lesbians, penal reform do-gooders, the Government have permitted a state of affairs where they have no views, no principles nor disciplines, and as a result, money pours from the national coffers for any purpose whatever and welfare spending runs out of control, grabbing a sixth of everything the nation produces.

The elderly feel that this Government is ready to listen to any pressure group but never to them, but the elderly have the power to change this state of affairs.

We are meant to live by the disciplines and principles imposed on our society by Church and Government but if they have no principles, anything goes. It is sad that a feckless Government is matched by a wimpish Church.

And following the approval of female clergy, the resulting crisis in the Anglican Church is another upset for the elderly churchgoer.   Whatever one's opinion might be, it is a fact that where the Church dominates and takes a strong moral line there are few unmarried mothers, and families care for their elderly.

The lone voice of the Pope is heard challenging the plague of divorce, and fiercely attacking safe sex. and the present chaos in much of sexual behaviour. With such an example of uncompromising moral leadership it is no wonder that five Church of England bishops lead an exodus of 570 clergymen from the CofE to Rome in protest at the appointment of women priests.

Most elderly were churchgoers at one time, but when you consider that active CofE congregations in the U.K. have fallen from 27 million to 1.1 million, that 300 churches have been demolished and 900 closed, all in the last 20 years there is obviously something wrong.

The wimpish hierarchy of the Church of England has done little but waffle, and it's failure to condemn such evils as homosexuality, even approving gay clergymen, was an absolute turn-off for many elderly. Only 15% of the population of the U.K. are active church members, a lower proportion than in any other European country.

Even in the current parliamentary vote for lowering the age of consent for homosexuals, the Anglican bishops are unable to agree, or to condemn it. Most elderly expect them to condemn it out of hand but some, Edinburgh and Monmouth even favour reducing the age to 16, others think 18, others 21. A free vote in Parliament decided to compromise at 18, as did the House of Lords, but where is the religious thunder of utter condemnation?

If sufficient influential voices had been raised the acknowledgment of queers, (why should they usurp the beautiful word 'gay'), and lesbian influence, both of which are totally abhorrent to the elderly, would have been condemned and suppressed as they should be.

A lesbian headmistress in the London Borough of Hackney prevented her 200 pupils from seeing the ballet Romeo and Juliet because she thought that the children in her control should be involved with 'all forms of sex'. Although it seems that the female chairman of the governors who appointed her to her £500 a week job just happened to be living with her as her lesbian lover, it transpired that she was doing well in a tough area. Her union protested that she was being hounded out of her job, since she was a member of Hackney Gay and Lesbian Teacher's Association. Well might the elderly exclaim, "What are we coming to?"

The Government, which must obviously take

ultimate responsibility for allowing queer headmasters and lesbian headmistresses, allows time to debate lowering the homosexual age of consent. That they should waste a single second of their time on such an unsavoury topic, is beyond the belief of most elderly.

To acknowledge queers at all illustrates this Government's lack of principle in paying regard to any cause, and in this particular case, despite recent proof that the strength of the queer's campaign is out of proportion to the numbers involved. The talented queers of ballet, theatre and the arts have spilled over into influencing what is shown on our television screens. The B.B.C. has a Lesbian and Gay Group which fought for a marriage allowance to be paid to a pair of homosexuals. This influence should be constantly monitored.

The fact that such creatures gain parliamentary time at all really stirs up the elderly, some of whom gave vent to their opinions as, "Homosexuality is wrong and should never have been legalised in the first place," "I was in the Navy and just to talk about queers makes my flesh creep," "queers should crawl back under the stones they came from and keep quiet about it," "they're sickening, they should be exterminated, it was about the only good thing Hitler did," "why give it a chance to spread when it is bad enough as it is," "I would ban homosexuality absolutely; it seems you can't stop it but why encourage it."

But this Government allows time for a debate and John Major, Prime Minister, allows time for a principal queer to visit him. Perhaps that obscenely disgusting practice of importuning in public lavatories will next receive the approval of Church and State, or is this supposed to be a different matter.

In the same week that the story broke about the 17-year young offender being sent on a £7,000 holiday by the special school in Wales, the South Wales police reported that they would have to close a large number of their 74 police stations through lack of money. Unless they had more money they would also lose 200 policemen and staff. Under Government capping regulations there was no more money for police.

The £1,800 a week that is spent for each boy would buy a few policemen and then there wouldn't be so much crime to have to pay for. Even in the matter of crime the Government must be doing something wrong somewhere because we have more prisoners locked up than in any other EU country. This table shows the population and the numbers in prison:-

U.K.	56,467,000	55,457
Germany	80,372.000	52,076
France	56,614,000	46,423
Italy	57,193,000	34,675
Spain	38,872,268	29,244
Portugal	10,582,000	8,181
Belgium	9,928,000	6,450
Netherlands	15,240,000	5,827
Greece	10,256,464	4,288

(In 1960 there were 26,824 prisoners in England and Wales)

The weekly cost per place and inmate varies according to the type of accommodation, from £816 per prisoner per week in Dispersal Prisons to £331 in Open Prisons. The average cost per prisoner is £494 per week. Your pocket calculator will tell you that 55,457, at £494 costs the country £27,395,758 a week, even half of which would give every pensioner another pound a week.

According to the 1994 Social Trends published by the Central Statistical Office, people from the black ethnic minority are eight times more likely to become prisoners than whites.

It is interesting to recall that up to the year 1800 there were no prisons; punishment was by the birch, flogging and capital punishment and there was no need for prisons.

The Government announce that they are going to get really tough on crime. A thug who smashes the frail body of an old lady is going to prison. But, of course, no physical harm will come to him. He will have three good meals a day so he'll never be hungry like the old lady might be, he'll be warm, too, not having to worry about VAT on fuel like she will, he'll have free TV, recreation, maybe a key to his own cell as they do in some prisons. His safety, comfort and welfare will be assured by do-gooders. A regime, so tough, in fact, that thugs commit the same crimes again and again with no fear whatever of the penalty that our feeble society will impose upon them, with no fear whatever of another cosy spell in prison.

A parliamentary written answer reveals:-

that 71% of Under-21 male prisoners re-offend

that 57% of male prisoners re-offend

that 54% of those doing Community Service re-offend

that 52% of prisoners on probation re-offend

that 51% of Under-21 female prisoners re-offend

that 40% of female prisoners re-offend

A report in the MERTHYR EXPRESS quotes a man just released from prison as saying that he wouldn't mind booking into prison for a relaxing month a year. He had a carpeted cell, three meals a day, satellite TV and video, his own cell key and freedom to go to bed and get up when he liked.

A MORI poll reports
that notifiable offences in England and Wales have risen in the last five years by 44% to nearly 5.6 million.
that 79%, and 89% in the North East, fear having their homes burgled
that 57% of women, (and 78% under age 25), fear being raped

that 67% of women are afraid to go out after dark

The number of cars stolen in England and Wales is more than double the European average and more than most countries in the world, as the following table shows:

Percentage of cars stolen each year

England and Wales ,,,................ 3.1%
Italy 3.0%
Australia 3/0%
New Zealand 2.8%
France 2.8%
USA 2.5%
Northern Ireland 2.2%
Sweden 2.0%
Spain 1.9%
Norway 1.3%
Poland 1.3%
Czechoslovakia 1.2%
Scotalnd 1.2%
Canada 1.2%
Belgium 1.1%
Japan 0.6%
Germany 0.5%
Holland 0.5%
Luxembourg 0.0%

CHAPTER SIX

We have lived through an era of mergers and takeovers, of great benefit to the community we were told, although the benefit was never made clear to the workers made redundant, nor to the shops and communities in areas surrounding factories closed, and quickly derelict.

Although there have always been companies joining forces on a modest scale, public attention was first directed to the takeover business when Charles Clore successfully bid for Freeman, Hardy and Willis and his method was subsequently adopted by others in the City. At the time there was more or less full employment in Britain.

After the Clore takeover, and into the 1960s, even the Labour Government of the time supported takeovers and mergers, believing that British industry was too fragmented to be able to compete with larger foreign rivals, and taking a benign view of the growth of takeovers in the hope of improving Britain's competitiveness in the world.

In 1967/68, Arnold Weinstock took over AEI and then merged with English Electric, cutting Head Office staff from 2,000 to 200 and closing thirtyfive branch headquarters. Profits then proceeded to treble, which was fine for Mr. (now Lord) Weinstock and the shareholders but not much comfort to all the workers he had sacked.

It so happened that, despite GEC becoming one of Britain's biggest companies, the U.K. productive share of electrical and electronic goods declined, unable to halt the flow of Japanese and European firms dominating the domestic market; so much so that GEC was soon forced to retire from making domestic appliances, TVs and radio.

We continued to witness wholesale closures and redundancies following the big takeovers and mergers of the 1960s and 1970s.

Following 20,000 takeovers and mergers in the United States there were, in Britain, 1,000 takeovers in one year, then 2,000 in less than a year.

In how many of these was a thought given to the effect of transferring responsibility for the livelihood of workers from private enterprise to the tax payer, quite apart from the domino effect of the loss of their buying power, and loss of local taxes from properties closed. Unfortunately, at this time, the Trade Unions were losing their influence and their power of protest.

Banks and merchant banks pushed customer companies to make takeover bids, more to give the banks takeover profits than for any other reason. Taking over businesses became a business in itself, a money trading game, banks and merchant banks set up special take-over departments which then needed to be employed despite charging astronomical fees for their services, services supposedly promoting the theory of market forces, but actually catering for greed, short term profit and megalomania.

The takeover trade was just figures with file names of companies, themselves simply commodities to be traded, bought and sold, their actual trade irrelevant as was the fate of their workers, tossed on to the unemployment scrapheap that these clever business games created. Hundreds of smart takeover advisers 'earned' more than £1 million a year by doing so, ending the working lives of millions. It demonstrated the working of the free market as it has been allowed to develop, but not how manufacturing industries survive.

The really great companies became great by fulfilling and expanding their original role, and not by patchworking ill assorted assets for the sake of greed and megalomania only.

The Government and the City showed little concern for the longer term implications, the destruction of the established job framework for ever. As for the financial implications, insider trading and dubious financial practices were suspected at the highest level, culminating in the infamous Guinness affair. This took untold millions in fees, advertising, backhanders and unsavoury manoeuvring in the City, to the extent that at last the Government developed misgivings about other excesses in the City of London, Lloyds scandals, the Johnson Mathey Bank collapse. As we all know there were many more unsavoury development to come. One of those named in the Guinness affair, Ivan Boesky, had earlier made over £20 million in a single deal involving the Nestlé takeover of Carnation. The principals involved in the Guinness affair were rightly jailed, but there were many on the fringe, an outer charmed circle of collaborators who sought to gain from a doubtful transaction.

Asset stripping was another dubious development. Not all the companies taken over by predators like Slater, Walker had fat and lazy managements nor did they need to have reserves raided with the excuse that dead assets were being liberated to be channelled into more successful enterprises, (successful for whom?).

If a firm was surviving on modest profits, providing

employment and security for its workers and the community, the predator who took it over, sacked half its workers and closed the premises, would be the principal person to gain.

Maybe many of the thousands of companies taken over were not operating at 100% efficiency, maybe they were not earning a reasonable return on capital employed, but what did that matter so long as they were surviving to provide employment and helping to keep communities intact.

It was inevitable that mechanization and computerization should result in jobs disappearing for ever, but the loss of jobs through greed and now, in recent years through policies of downsizing could surely be critically examined, particularly if it is workers who are losing their jobs and bureaucrats retained.

Companies are being allowed to shed tens of thousands of jobs, at enormous cost to the taxpayer, without any evidence of Government concern for the consequences.

The clearing banks will be shedding 100,000 jobs we are told. Privatised public utilities, like electricity and water, shed jobs but at the same time pay millions to mediocre bosses.

Unless a Government seeks to control the number of workers discarded by private enterprise solely for reasons of profit or greed, so will the jobs-lost-for-ever increase, the burden on the taxpayer spiralling down to the economic collapse of the country.

As for those who depend upon the State pension for survival, it is time to realise that we older folk have the voting power to influence our future, we have the power to stop others from manipulating the chess game of our lives and treating us as the pawns we are at the moment.

It is difficult to believe that once upon a time there were over 300 companies manufacturing sprodgets in this country. The average price of a sprodget was £2.50 and they were consistent in shape and quality whoever made them.

Then, maybe thirty or so years ago, Bristol Sprodgets bought out Wiltshire Sprodgets, closed the Wiltshire premises in a market town just outside of Salisbury, and moved production to Bristol. Only 651 people lost their jobs at Salisbury, the premises stayed empty and the knock-on effect of loss to the community was very sad. In fact, some time later, the ex-owner of Wiltshire Sprodgets was sad, too, when he saw how many of his loyal ex-workers were still redundant, and how desolate his still empty factory looked, with shops round that had been dependant on him, desolate too. He realised that he could easily have gone on trading in a modestly successful way, keeping his family of employees together and the community, and himself also, for all he had now to fill his empty days was the money that had tempted him to sell.

This one takeover heralded a rash of others. Bristol Sprodgets went on to take over Surrey, Lancs, East Yorkshire, Durham, Macclesfield and Dagenham Sprodgets with encouragement and major funding from commercial banks. Altogether seventeen factories were closed and a total workforce of 4,680 was reduced to 1,360, yet achieving the same output of sprodgets. It was a magnificient achievement.

There could be no stopping such progress and the flotation of Bristol Sprodgets was a memorable success on the Stock Market. Other sprodget companies fell like ninepins before its triumphant advance.

When he achieved his 100th takeover, the owner of Bristol Sprodgets was knighted, and received a congratulatory visit from the Lady Prime Minister at his new factory. Government policy encouraged such bold industrial enterprise. With a streamlined workforce of 7,670 he was now producing as many sprodgets as had previously been produced in one hundred factories by over a million workers.

"This is the sort of achievement that the country needs," said the PM is a moving speech.

The rest of the story is well known. There are now

only two sprodget manufacturers in the whole country. Nobody can do without sprodgets, of course, and although the price of a sprodget has gone up to £29.99, spokespersons for these two monopoly manufacturers are quick to reassure us, to deny that they use their monopoly position to screw suppliers into the ground and to fix selling prices at an artifically high level.

The Bristol Sprodgets owner who started it all is now Lord Sprodget and is said to be worth £600 million. A member of his family is well placed in Government.

In view of his enormously successful experience the PM has asked him for his help with the Government problem of unemployment, not to mention the serious loss of tax revenue from various sources. Also keenly sought by the Government are his views on how to avoid the problem of cities and towns and villages where derelict factories and shops are such a depressing feature for the communities who live there.

Unfortunately, Lord Sprodget was not able to devote much time to this because foreign made sprodgets were providing fierce competition. He was able to maintain the profitability level of the company by making 540 workers redundant. In the end, competitive pressure became too great and Lord Sprodget sold out to the Japanese for £400 million.

A carping critic in the House was roundly condemned when he complained that the actions of Lord Sprodget had resulted in three quarters of a million unemployed and the closure of two hundred and eighty factories, creating an enormous burden on the taxpayer with the sole result of achieving vast wealth for Lord Sprodget and his family.

Such defeatist talk was not in the best interests of the country said the PM in another moving speech, in which she declared that Britain needed the introduction of foreign capital.

Although our elderly generation has lived through much of a century of progress unmatched in history, from horse travel to supersonic, from before telephones and wireless sets to talking to outer space, for most old people today, modern living does not compare with yesterday.

We have seen much of the convenience of life disappear in the name of progress. We remember when almost everybody had shops nearby for all we needed. We remember grocer's shops, for instance, with long, polished wood counters, in front of which there were bentwood chairs for customers while being served or waiting.

Everything you wanted was placed before you on the counter, maybe your wishes and your name were known. Tastings were offered and the whole business was a little social occasion, friendly, with the final, "Shall we put in on the account?" and "We will deliver your order this afternoon."

One thousand seven hundred local sub-post offices have closed despite the enormous convenience they afforded. The greater efficiency claimed to have been achieved by their closure is not apparent to the 20,000 or so elderly folk, each having to walk another mile or so every week to collect their pension.

The elderly have seen the virtual disappearnce of

convenience local retailers, killed by the impact of competition from out of town superstores. Not only are the few remaining traditional neighbourhood shops suffering through lack of custom but they cannot buy from suppliers on the same terms as those demanded by supermarkets. Small shops close down, towns and villages that once sparkled with the charm of multiple trades now fade in the gloom of shuttered, empty shops, only relieved by window displays of interminable and boring building societies. Now, we read, out-of-town shopping centres are to be curbed to protect the traditional British high street. The quality of life in town and cities is to be protected. Is it unfair to suggest that this is yet another instance of the Government realising too late the results of their policies, or lack of them. They are only stirred to plan the closure of stable doors by the clatter of horse's hooves galloping away.

Despite this pathetic example of stern Government resolve, Sainsburys and Safeway still announce their plans to open 20 new stores a year as though they are a law unto themselves as well they well might be. It seems that plans for 400 new stores have already been approved.

How we should all rejoice if local shops crept back again and we all supported them, and High Streets glowed with life and local trade again, and all the out of town superstores withered and died. Alas for such hopes. Although the worst effects of monopolies, takeovers and mergers might, with some forethought, have been avoided, technological progress, the effects of micro-technology, for instance, have sounded the death knell for many jobs since the 1980s.

In 1979 there were 10,000 industrial robots in the world, (compared to 4,000 in 1975), mostly in the U.S. and Japan, although there were 500 in France. Before General Motors took on robots they were building sixty cars an hour; with welding robots they were building one hundred cars an hour. They found that robots never tire, never miss work but, as General Motors also discovered, they have one enormous disadvantage. They don't buy motorcars.

When we progress to the point that all the work of the world could be done by robots and computers, who will there be to buy? Who will there be to pay taxes?

We experienced the exciting emerging days of motoring, the Austin 7 and the Morris 8.

In our day, roads were mercifully free of motorcars and few of us owned them in the early years. With their posh, modern tech cars the younger generation wouldn't know what a starting handle looked like but at least, when we were able to afford a car, we knew the joy of the really open road, parking right outside places that we wished to visit whether seaside, country, London, anywhere.

Whatever progress has been achieved, there is no doubt that we enjoyed the best days of motoring, British motoring and pride in a breathtaking selection of magic marques, all different in character and style, Lea-Francis, Humber, Bean, Calcott, Standard, Wolseley, Armstrong-Siddeley, Clyno, Crossley, Lanchester, Riley, Singer, Trojan.

Whose fault was it that this great U.K. industry declined until we reached the stage of being grateful to the Japanese, our once proud car makers having to depend upon Japanese technology and design for survival. And now Rover, Britain's last indigenous mass car producer has been taken over by the German BMW, the once great British motor industry that challenged the world in our time, lost to foreign ownership, and Japanese and German at that.

William Morris and Herbert Austin must be revving in their graves.

Through all the years of our decline, the French car industry has survived with Renault, Peugeot, Citroen. The German car industry has survived with Mercedes, BMW, Volkswagen, the Italians with Fiat, Alfa Romeo, the Swedes with Volvo, Saab etc.

And while they are all surviving, maybe with Government help and subsidy, the British car industry created by the founding fathers of motoring, is wiped out, from which you can only assume that there is something wrong with our leadership and guidance. Where is the wisdom at the helm?

And while you are pausing and reflecting on the sad history of the British motor industry during our lifetime, spare even sadder thoughts for those magic names of our youth, Norton, Velocette, Matchless, Ariel, Triumph, Douglas, A.J.S., Scott, Sunbeam, BSA, Royal Enfield.

Somebody, somewhere has got a lot to answer for.

Fine, old established shipyards and their skilled workers are allowed to rot while we permit British shipping companies to have their new ships built in Germany. One of the greatest names, Swan Hunter, is about to be taken over by the French.

We remember trains. Clutching tightly a parent's hand, on the station amidst the luggage, spellbound at the magic approach of a vast, green, snorting engine, sighing fierce clouds of steam in all directions as though raging at his little oily driver for daring to stop him at a station. Opening the door straight into the carriage, black and white pictures of the resort you were going to, friendly porters in their sleeved waistcoats actually carrying your luggage and putting it on the rack for you.

In 1957 there were 17,527 steam engines and by 1968 that number had been reduced to 362.

In the early 1960s we remember Dr. Beeching being authorised by the Government to discover which passenger and freight services were making a profit.

He found that one third of route miles carried 1% of passenger traffic and 1.5% of freight. Just 118 stations out of 2,067 were dealing with 52% of freight traffic carried.

As a result, 5,000 route miles out of a total of 18,214 were closed as were a third of all passenger stations.

The Beeching Plan dealt with making the railways profitable, without regard for social need, and without regard for a national transport plan with linking roles for rail and road. Today, our rail network is unsatisfactory and our roads are clogged with heavy traffic, much of which should be carried by rail.

How interesting to see that the Swiss voted recently to ban large foreign lorries from their country, insisting that the goods should be carried by rail, to the obvious benefit of both rail and road. How lucky the Swiss are to be allowed to have a say in what they want by way of a referendum. It will be remembered that the Swiss voted against membership of the European Free Trade area and are no worse for having done so.

We remember coal fires and all the conflict and bitterness about closing coal mines, after nationalisation in 1946 had promised such high hopes for the mining communities.

There are many elderly in the mining villages, existing now amidst the misery created by widespread unemployment, shuttered shops, fifty men chasing every job advertised, and worse to come.

During the recent crisis regarding the closure of even more British coal mines, an elderly lady showed me a bag of coal that had been delivered to her; it was marked 'Produced in Germany.' It was revealed that we were importing electricity from France, equivalent to the output of five pits, the cross-channel electricity flowing into Britain along a £1 billion cable from Calais to a National Grid converter station at Sellindge, near Folkestone.

It seems that British electricity users are paying a hidden subsidy of £150 million a year which is helping to keep French miners in work. Imagine the outcry there would be in France if the situation was reversed.

If the regional supply companies took electricity produced by Britain's coal fired power stations, some of our pits could be saved. And who decided that Aldermaston atomic weapons factory in Berkshire is to be fuelled by Russian coal. How must redundant miners in North Staffordshire feel when their free coal allowance is delivered to them by British Coal - from Poland.

Although it is a fact that British pits produce the cheapest deep mined coal in Europe, with production costs half those of Germany, two-thirds those of Spain and three-quarters those of France, the British Government still buys subsidised coal from abroad.

Apparently the British taxpayer has invested £12 billion in our coal industry in the last twenty years and now this Government is proposing to throw all this away, even now deciding to hand over mines to private enterprise.

It seems that nuclear power stations are built despite the fact that we don't need any more power stations at all. The amount of taxpayers' money spent on subsiding the nuclear power industry is equal to a subsidy of £50 per tonne for British coal - solving the British miner's problems and benefiting the country at the same time, not to mention avoiding the possibility of a Chernobyl disaster in this country.

The current crazy idea of the Government to close another thirtyone pits, will decimate the lives of one hundred thousand miners and their families. This

Government has set aside £1 billion for redundancies alone, just half of which would keep all the thirtyone pits open. This is fact, not an opinion.

We have seen some of the mistakes made by this Government and, with coal, they are about to make another of massive proportions even for them. There is widespread sympathy for the miners amongst the elderly, who wish that they could do something. Maybe we can.

We remember tramcars, wind-up gramophones and toasting forks. We remember Lyon's tea shops, meeting at Corner Houses during the war.

We remember when dance bands played music, with lyrics singing of love, not sex:-

> *Some day he'll come along*
> *The man I love,*
> *And he'll be big and strong,*
> *The man I love;*
> *And when he comes my way,*
> *I'll do my best to make him stay.*
> *He'll look at me and smile,*
> *I'll understand;*
> *And in a little while*
> *He'll take my hand;*
> *And though it seems absurd,*

I know we both won't say a word.
Maybe I shall meet him Sunday,
Maybe Monday maybe not;
Still I'm sure to meet him one day,
Maybe Tuesday will be my good news day.
He'll built a little home,
Just meant for two,
From which I'll never roam,
Who would, would you?
And so all else above,
I'm waiting for the man I love.

We remember when we could wander home from dances, full of dreams, clutching our dancing shoes in a paper bag, happy and safe however late.

We remember when armchairs faced each other around the fire, when we spoke to each other in the evenings, were aware of each other, read, sewed, played music.

THE ELDERLY ARE BEING DENIED THE COMPLETE NATIONAL HEALTH SERVICE THAT THEY DESERVE

(There is discrimination in the Health Service against old people because of the need to ration resources)

CHAPTER SEVEN

If we don't use our Elderly voting power to vote for ourselves there won't be a National Health Service left for the Elderly at all.

When you reach pension age you need to realise that the National Health Service is not 100% for you any more. The Health Service is not available to you as a right any more but only if services happen to be available. *Unless you use your voting power to form an ELDER PARTY you will be dealt with medically not according to your need but according to your life expectancy.*

Too much money has been, and is being wasted in other directions and the elderly, the most deserving section of the community, are now last in the Health

Service queue.

When you realise that we, the elderly, represent the largest potential voting group in the country you should be moved to vote for your age group, for the ELDER PARTY, so that we can influence a better deal for ourselves.

Having put up with poor pensions and poor conditions is something that one gradually becomes used to, but when you start getting turned down for medical treatment you have a real problem. Imagine being really ill and being turned away by a hospital just because you are old. Don't think that this couldn't happen to you because, according to the Royal College of Physicians it is happening now.

But we can make sure that the Health Service looks after us and puts us first in the queue. The power of voting strength is in our hands.

The Royal College of Physicians report, (May 1994), that elderly people are regularly being refused life-saving surgery and medical treatment, not because of their medical condition but because of their age.

One in five Coronary Care Departments discriminated against pensioners who needed emergency heart treatment, and four out of ten were refused life-saving drugs after a heart attack. Coronary Care units may not admit someone over 75.

Elderly patients were often denied treatment for

kidney dialysis and transplant surgery.

We need to be considered on the basis of medical need, not age, and admission to hospital should be decided on need, not age; access to specialist facilities should be equally available to the elderly.

But researchers found that 20% of Coronary Care Units refused to treat patients over age 70; that one in five Coronary Care units imposed age limits on patients they would treat, and that four out of ten refused to give clot busting drugs to older people.

This situation has arisen because of the Government lack of resources, because of waste on a vast scale.

Over the years we came to have regard for the National Health Service, and it does not seem long ago that you could feel confident of receiving hospital treatment when you wanted it.

The NHS has been allowed to decline, and the whole system has become so inefficient, wasteful and costly that it is not only undermining its chances of survival but threatening the availability of resources for the Elderly.

The size of hospital waiting lists has come to be regarded as the modern barometer of NHS efficiency.

In addition, care of the elderly has deteriorated since the Government Care in the Community reforms were introduced, according to the British

Medical Association. Elderly residents are heartlessly turned out of homes in which they had hoped to spend the rest of their days, "to give the best service." Doctors were finding it harder to get help for elderly patients, and it had become more difficult for patients who could not look after themselves to get into a nursing home.

The BMA criticism was based on the opinions of 85% of doctors. A junior health minister said that care in the community had made a good start. Who would you be inclined to believe?

It is not as though the vast amounts spent, and wasted, do anything to improve efficiency.

The Royal College of Surgeons report that in four out of ten hospitals, surgeons have been told to slow down the number of operations they perform because their hospital is running out of money.

If your doctor now happens to be a new-style fund-holding GP you will be able to jump the queue for hospital treatment, according to the British Medical Association. Fund holding doctors apparently have more money than health authorities, but even this is now subject to the age of the patient.

The BMA organised a survey of doctors and found that four in ten hospitals allowed patients of fund-holding doctors to jump queues for treatment.

However much the Government may deny it, it is

a fact that a large number of elderly people have surgery deferred because of the inability of the NHS to treat them through lack of money. Because of Government incompetence and waste there are not enough resources available to look after the health of the elderly. *Older people are being denied treatment in the U.K. that is available to pensioners of similar age and condition in other European countries.*

The situation is apparently going to get worse as people get older and Government incompetence reduces money available.

The situation will most certainly get worse unless we, the elderly, use the power of our voting numbers to do something about it. If we don't, medical resources will be increasingly allocated not according to need but according to a patient's life expectancy, and this is happening in ever increasing numbers at the moment.

It is all very well the Government claiming that the NHS was available for everybody, whatever their age, but this was not being borne out in practice according to the knowledgable opinion of the Royal College of Physicians.

Medical opinion confirms that there is discrimination in the NHS against old people because of the need to ration resources.

Since lack of money is the cause of NHS failure, it

is obviously the fault of the Government in failing to anticipate and provide, not to mention executive and financial incompetence in seeking to provide. The Royal College of Nursing report that patients are being forced to wait overnight for a bed in almost one in three accident and emergency units. The NHS has lost 121,000 beds in just over ten years; 10,600 beds were closed last year.

Where has all the money gone?

The bill for social security has risen by half in the last three years. In three months the Government paid out £21.9 billion in pensions, housing benefit, invalidity benefit, family credit and sickness payments. This is obviously a rate of spending that cannot be sustained, but do we ever question the competence or qualifications of the minister allowed to be in charge of such vast amounts of our money. Would any business allow such ill qualified people to be in charge of the petty cash department.

Even before the various worthy causes can seek their share of the National Cake, Government incompetence limits the amount available.

For instance, they allow the Wessex Health Authority to waste £43 million of taxpayers money on a computer project which had to be abandoned.

In 1993 the NHS bill for staff cars increased from £53 million to £70 million. In the new Trust hospitals the staff car bill rose from £5.3 million to £24 million.

It is understandable that District Nurses should have a car as part of their job but why should senior managers, who get well paid enough anyhow, have superior and costly cars as a perk. To quote but one example, the newly combined Guy's and St. Thomas's Trust in South London has 31 executive cars provided purely as perks for managers. You would imagine that these NHS executives were paid enough to be able to afford their own cars. Specimen salaries were £37,000, (£711 a week), £66,000, (£1,269 a week), £92,507, (£1,778 a week), £97,000, (£1,865 a week) and even one of £137,000, (£2,634 per week), all having had 8.7% increases in the last financial year

Government reforms of the NHS, for instance, intended to reduce the appalling delays that the elderly, and others, have to endure, produced 1,500 more administrators over three years but only 50 more doctors, and this was in Wales alone.

They have also created a complete absence of financial responsibility. Two managers travelled to the United States by Concorde for the week end at a cost of £8,500.

In England the salary bill for hospital managers rose, between 1986 and 1992, from eleven million to four hundred and ninetyfour million. The number of managers rose from one thousand to thirteen thousand two hundred but the number of nurses rose by only three thousand.

A new NHS hotline to deal with information cost £1.4 million, (average cost £22 per call), a total amount of money that would have enabled 233 hip operations to be carried out.

And with all this change and reorganisation and so-called improvement, hospital beds are vanishing and hospitals have to make desperate efforts to find beds at other hospitals for acutely ill patients, and other patients, many of whom are elderly, wait, often in pain or inconvenience. Next day admissions are routinely cancelled and operations deferred. These facts are based on complaints by the doctors involved.

Even famous hospitals are closed against the wishes and advice of the doctors concerned. The transfer of medical services from Guy's to St. Thomas's prompted Guy's consultants to say, "Many more Londoners will now be convinced that the NHS is not safe in this Government's hands." At the centre of the row it was claimed that a £140 million high-tech unit would become a white elephant.

The amount of money spent on clerks and managers in the first National Health Hospital Trust doubled in the first two years, from £2.4 million to £4.2 million, and nearly a million had to be transferred from care of patients to the cost of bureaucrats.

Under National Health Trusts, bureaucracy has soared. Not only have the number of managers risen from 1,230 to 14,980 in four years but many enjoy palatial offices. The new £55 million headquarters of the National Health Management Executive in Leeds has a heated swimming pool, sports hall and a £14,000 hand woven carpet in the foyer.

Scandals of bureaucratic waste and inefficiency in setting up NHS Trusts are to be curbed by the Health Minister, (she says), but what the elderly want to know, is why she allowed them to happen in the first place. £70 million has been spent by the Trust Hospitals in advertising their new services.

Prescription cheats are allowed to cost the NHS £30 million a year.

Criticisms of the Health Department come from the people who know, the people involved. A retiring NHS Trust chairman complained that there were managers to negotiate with new managers, accountants to negotiate with accountants, marketing people that have never been seen. Figures from the Department of Health itself show a 30,000 increase in managers, clerical and administrative staff in the last four years.

In the West Midlands Regional Health Authority, 1,555 hospital beds were withdrawn during 1991,1992.

An all party committee of MPs found that this Health Authority had wasted £10 million, enough to pay for 20,000 beds or 880 junior nurses for a year

At Gloucestershire Royal Hospital fifty cars are leased at a cost of £2,500 a year each, £125,000 a year and that is just one hospital. Multiply that for the country and it is no wonder that the elderly are deprived to pay for all this profligacy.

Bureaucrats, supposedly overseeing local NHS services, appointed management consultants at an unauthorised fee of £4 million. Government weaknesses in management and accountability were discovered. Nevertheless, the chairman of the disgraced regional authority retired with a golden handshake of £10,000. The director of Regionally Managed Services was, after five years, given lump sums totalling £81,000 and an immediate pension of £124 a week.

With the revolution in the NHS structure dividing up into separate accountable businesses, they run into difficulties if they happen to have in their area a patient needing vital, but expensive drugs, sometimes costing as much as a million pounds over a year. Previously, such exceptional cases would form only a small part of the national budget but now, in order to meet the cost from a small budget, somebody has to go without.

Rationing of medical treatment by age is morally wrong, but the question of rationing would not arise at all if so much money was not wasted.

The number of managers in the London area of the Health Service has risen by the same number as nurses have been reduced. Staff are reduced but still costs rise. It is not as though the employment of more bureaucrats has freed doctors from form filling, to be able to concentrate on medical care; there are more meetings and committees and forms to be filled, the more bureaucrats are appointed to perpetuate this idiocy. We are now told that the number of bureaucrats is being reduced but why were they allowed in the first place. A third of the medical costs in the United States are attributable to the bureaucratic cost of estimating them.

Once upon a time there was a hospital and it dealt successfully and happily with about 1,000 patients a week.

One day it was decided that the hospital ought to have a manager so one was appointed at a moderate salary of £1,000 a week. Naturally he needed staff but he limited this to only twentynine and there was no problem in finding them suitable offices because there was a ward that could be converted at a nominal cost of £450,000. The sixteen old ladies who had been looked after comfortably in the ward were re-located into the community, thus maintaining the splendid average of turning old people out of hospital care, the bed numbers having fallen from 51,000 to 37,500 being cared for in only five years.

The manager and his staff were needed to put into force the clever new Purchaser/Provider bureaucratic NHS system where looking after patients had to be arranged by contracts, between doctors and hospitals, hospitals and health authorities. Patients were to become business units to be bargained for, so he invented a lot of clever forms that he sent round to doctors and nurses for them to fill in. This was no problem because they could easily turn away a few patients each day so that they could fill up their forms and the manager expanded his managing.

From form filling he moved on to organising meetings and these were soon so successful that he was able to have them in the mornings and afternoons. There were morning meetings with consultants to make sure that they were explaining what they would be doing, rather than doing it, and another morning to examine the cost of what they would be doing if they weren't prevented from doing it by being at the meeting, and several meetings a week on management committees, weekly meetings about medical accounts and other meetings to establish what they were doing with their time. The consultants and doctors and nurses who had to attend these meetings were able to do so by cancelling appointments and operations so that no difficulties were created. Since one in five coronary care departments in the NHS were discriminating against people of pension age, the manager was able to follow suit, also refusing life saving drugs after such patients had had a heart attack; according to the Royal College of Physicians this was happening in four out of ten hospitals anyhow and the money saved allowed the upgrading of senior manager's cars. In fact, for every £1 spent on patient care, only £3.50 was spent on the bureaucrats who organised it so that the system was obviously working splendidly.

The manager became so busy that additional staff were needed to keep records of what his staff were doing and it was a simple matter to locate them since office accommodation could be created for only £600,000 by converting one of the theatres that had been used for kidney dialysis but the surgeons were now too busy attending committee meetings and, in any case, it brought the hospital into line with other hospitals that were treating far fewer such patients than hospitals in Europe despite similar levels of disease.

Dealing with doctors created another form filling opportunity, (when the doctors could spare the time from their extensive form filling activities, without which they weren't paid). Doctors had to ask the hospital if suitable contracts existed and if the required treatment had been negotiated and who would pay for it and was an appeal likely.

To simplify proceedings the manager closed another ward to instal a major computer system at a bargain cost of £43 million; and now, at the touch of a button, the speed at which they were able to cancel appointments and operations was most impressive. And with this computer it only took seven weeks of administration to organise one and a half hours of treatment which again proved the value of the new system. The clerical and administrative work necessary to produce the statistics for star ratings for the performance of hospitals naturally took preference over the patient care in the hospital

So successful was the manager and all his additional staff that the total numbers of people attending the hospital was cut from the original 1,000 a week to only 300, and they received a letter from the Lady Minister congratulating them upon their achievement.

To further improve efficiency it was decided to close this hospital as a hospital and convert it entirely to an administrative centre for the benefit of other hospitals in the area. The cost of providing salaries and benefits and motor vehicles for administrative staff had reached the stage where the budget could only be balanced by cutting out the health service; but the hospital had catered mainly for elderly people who were not qualifying for so much health consideration now because they had less life expectancy.

The merging of hospitals increased NHS efficiency. Although the hospital had been established for a hundred years, creating a specialist reputation, it would not entail any inconvenience to the elderly patients who attended for regular treatment because their age was disqualifying them for a number of treatments anyhow, and for the treatments still available to them there was an ever widening range of treatments just around the corner, only fourteen miles away.

Our need to prevent further deterioration of the National Health Service is urgent. Following the criticisms of the Bishop of Birmingham, the Chairman of the British Medical Association spoke of doctors in despair about what has been their place in a treasured national institution.

"Business plans," he said, "override clinical priority. Money does not follow the patient, the patient has no choice but to follow the money until it runs out." He spoke of the pernicious policies of local pay bargaining and privatisation of clinical support services, and of imposing performance related pay on hospital doctors.

He told his audience of doctors that there was no longer one unified Health Service but one hundred purchasing bodies and four hundred hospitals.

The conference he was addressing was made up of doctors, many senior, who showed that they agreed with the BMS Chairman's criticisms by giving him a standing ovation. How can it be, one wonders, that a Health Secretary with five years bureaucratic experience of the N.H.S. presumes to know better than the whole of the medical profession, all of whom are critical of the bureaucratic changes that they see affecting the care of you and me, their patients.

CHAPTER EIGHT

Where else does the money go?

In April 1994 it was reported that the Government had appointed consultants at a cost of £565 million to organise an efficiency drive which had resulted in the saving of £10 million.

Many elderly are understandably bewildered by the vast amounts awarded to women as a result of so called sexual discrimination. A policewoman was awarded £32,500 because she was not promoted to detective work. A £7,500 contribution to her costs was met by the Equal Opportunities Commission and the Commission for Racial Equality, and you don't need three guesses to know where their money came from, at the same time wondering just how much of the taxpayer's money goes to the grasping lawyers, who are allowed to hover like vultures over dubious opportunities. The Commission for Racial Equality is very noisy on behalf of its small percentage of the population. Most elderly strongly object, though privately, to the presumption of these people; if they choose to accept the hospitality of this country, not to mention DSS handouts and housing, they should conform to our customs and rules, and certainly not have the effrontery to expect us to defer to theirs. "When in Rome" etc. They generate publicity about ethnic minorities being disadvantaged - what about the millions of elderly who are disadvantaged, and nobody speaks up for them.

The deprived elderly are quietly outraged that ethnic minorities attract a far higher proportion of attention than their numbers warrant. The plight of coloured people in need is highlighted, but the plight of elderly people in need is not. Even a simple comment like this is immediately branded as racist, such is the hysteria generated by the vociferous ethnic minority groups.

If we can have a Commission for Racial Equality on behalf of 3,015,000 ethnic people in this country we most certainly ought to have a Commission for Elderly Equality on behalf of over eleven million elderly.

To speak for them, the Commission for Racial Equality has a chairman and deputy chairman and eleven members and a chief executive.

Ethnic minorities gained more time on television than their numbers in society justified. 7.4% of T.V. characters were of ethnic minorities but they only form 5.55% of the population.

In Birmingham there is a race relations team with a budget of £800,000.

The Equal Opportunities Commission head office is in Manchester and they have a Press Office in London, plus branch offices in Glasgow, Cardiff and Ireland. The lady chairman gets £604 a week and her deputy gets £540 a week and there are ten members and a chief executive.

A woman dismissed from the RAF for becoming pregnant was awarded £62,000. Another ex-RAF pregnant female was awarded £172,000 and it was estimated that tribunals were considering 2,200 similar cases. Settlements totalling £10 million have already been made, and the Ministry of Defence has accepted liability in a further 5,700 cases. An Army captain was awarded £24,000 and a former RAF woman received £33,000. Does anyone ever question whether such sums are really available to be paid, where it will come from, whether others, such as pensioners, will have to go short as a result of making such vast payments.

A former Wren who became pregnant was awarded £69,000 for unfair dismissal and sexual discrimination. Another was awarded £143,000. One would imagine that the Armed Forces was not a suitable occupation for a pregnant woman, nor for one with a small child;

that a woman who joined a fighting force automatically disqualified herself by becoming pregnant. And what are disabled, be-medalled ex-Service war heroes, men disabled for life in real action, now elderly and living on a pittance to make of a Government that can't find them another £1 a week but can easily discover in excess of £100,000 for any number of fit, ex-Service females who have earned it not in war but on their backs.

The endless payouts that we hear about are bad enough; but you can bet your life that for every example of wasteful incompetence we hear of there will be a dozen that we don't. The Ministry of Defence, for example is estimated to be paying an extra £25 to £30 million to contractors through failure to observe its own guidelines, according to the National Audit Office.

We are the only European country to give income support, housing benefit and council tax benefit without applying any test. £850 a month to a Lebanese, £500 a month to an Italian. Why not? The way our system is run it seems to be a soft touch for everybody except the needy, and particularly the elderly.

The Social Security budget of £80 billion must be cut, and since the Basic State Pension takes 1/3rd of it the elderly are in the firing line..

At the same time as all the NHS appalling waste is going on, the Social Services Secretary declared that "the one sure way to undermine the Welfare State would be to allow it to outstrip the nation's ability to pay, to expand without restraint," just as though some external agency unnconnected with his Government was responsible for the unbelievable waste of taxpayer's money.

It seems that there are unlimited amounts of money available for everybody except the old and it is certainly time that the elderly did something about it.

Already the Over 65s are being discriminated against in the matter of health care. This is fact, confirmed by the various professional medical organisations. As matters stand at the moment, you might have served your country when your country needed you, but now that you are old it is more than likely that when you need health service and care your country will have other things to do with the money available.

The Chief Secretary to the Treasury said that the Government had taken on too many roles that previously were left to welfare societies. In saying that the Government had taken on too many roles, this implies something that the Government have done in the past and are now correcting, some money saving lessons learnt, perhaps. One wonders if they know what money management means in the sense that businesses and households have to understand it. It is not difficult to understand why the Government has no more money available for pensions, for the elderly welfare and health care when you see how they allow taxpayer's money to be wasted in all directions. Taxpayers assets, like Chatham and Sheerness Docks are sold for £30 million to private owners who promptly sell them on for £108 million, a loss to you and me of £70 million. Can you imagine any private company allowing such idiocy?

An old lady suggested that times were hard for everybody, that perhaps the financial problems are so severe that our MPs are suffering the same hardship that we, the Elderly, are. If so, it would be unfair to accuse them of neglecting us if their money worries are piling up for them, also.

It is interesting to examine, therefore *by how much have MPs voted themselves salary increases compared to the increases they have provided for Retired folk:-*

THIS IS THE WEEKLY INCREASE THAT MPs HAVE VOTED FOR THEMSELVES NOT THE SALARY	THIS IS THE WEEKLY INCREASE THAT MPs HAVE VOTED FOR SINGLE PENSIONS
1980 44.23 weekly increase	3.85
1981 42.30 weekly increase	NIL
1982 10.76 weekly increase	2.45
1983 15.94 weekly increase	3.25
1984 15.34 weekly increase	1.20
1985 15.34 weekly increase	4.25
1986 15.34 weekly increase	.40
1987 15.34 weekly increase	.80
1988 77.84 weekly increase	1.65
1989 29.98 weekly increase	2.45
1990 49.88 weekly increase	3.30
1991 43.63 weekly increase	5.10
1992 36.23 weekly increase	4.37
1994 16.01 weekly increase	1.23
1995 16.32 weekly increase	

(the current increases are at the rate of 5.4% although inflation is at 1.8% and ministers are seeking to freeze Public Sector pay)
MPs pensions are 1/50th of salary for each year of service up to age 65 with a maximum of 2/3rds salary, or **£395.57 per week.**
But MPs have more expenses than you and I and therefore need higher salaries. Indeed? MPs get an Office Allowance of **£776.53 per week in addition to their salaries.**

And if pensioners today think that they are hard done by, the present Government is indicating that it wants people in future years to make their own provision for their own retirement, moving towards a situation where the State will not provide a pension at all.

Other financial advantages and sinecures abound by way of parliamentary consultancies.

It seems that the National Cake, which is unable to spare a big enough slice for the old, has an icing of gold available only for the privileged few.

And what are they doing for this country, these privileged few. Leadership has never been more needed and never less likely to emerge, unless we do something about using our voting strength to effect change.

A recent Gallup poll asked, "What will life hold for me next year?", (1994), to which only 11% of voters thought that their situation would improve. If this is true of a general cross section of the population what does the future hold for the elderly? It is in our hands to do something about it. It is in our hands to get some MPs of our own, a party of our own.

Quangos, (quasi autonomous non-governmental organisations), are growing in numbers again. There may be almost 2,000 of these 'jobs for the boys', costing the taxpayer £12 billion a year.

Will the waste of public money ever end under this Government? The revelation by a District Auditor of a Westminster Council scandal in which £21 million was allegedly lost by gerrymandering, is followed by the Public Accounts Committee making public a new catalogue of twenty financial failures and details of mismanagements. This report was made by an all party committee of MPs so there can be no question of political bias or motivation. It was the first time that the Committee had produced such a critical report in its history of 133 years. Sums like £80 million, £48 million, £11 million, £65 million were found to have been lost or wasted by various Government departments.

Can you imagine the remotest outpost of a multinational company, like ICI, being allowed to waste money, or to spend money as they please on anything that was not in accordance with strictly controlled company policy. Isn't it time we put in charge of this country people who have gained business experience and, at the same time, people who would realise the needs of the Elderly.

In our lifetime we have seen mismanagement of the nation's resources on a vast scale, with the result that now, in the most important years of our lives, we are likely to be last in the queue whichever party is in power.

So why not do something about it? Why not realise the strength of our numbers and have our own party, the Elder Party, to put our interests first in the queue, and the interests of the country in the hands of people with experience, wisdom and understanding.

ALTHOUGH THIS BOOK IS AIMED PRINCIPALLY AT OLDER FOLK, 65 AND OVER, THE OVER 55s WOULD CERTAINLY BENEFIT FROM THE FORMING OF AN ELDERLY PARTY.

CHAPTER NINE

Too old at 55?

At age 55 you may think it premature to be classed as Elderly; but from a driving point of view, according to the A.A., 55 is the youngest age at which medical research shows that our physical reactions begin to slow down.

Special holidays are offered to Over 55s and Over 55s are the target of insurance companies who offer you better terms because of your age. However much you may resent being considered different from a 45-year old, it seems that you are different.

In this computerised age, when employers shed staff in large numbers, the Over 55s are the first to go and are the least likely to be employed again. If Over 55s are out of work today they are never likely to find a job again if present conditions are allowed to continue.

The percentage of Over 55s in work today is only 45% compared to 70% in the pre-computer days.

Yet a newly appointed director, (over 60), of a national company commented on the absence of grey heads amongst the staff that he was meeting nationwide, the absence of experience.

If you are out of work at around age 50, whatever your experience or character, there is also a new reason why you may never work again; it is called Ageism, which seems to be discrimination against a person solely on account of age.

There are well publicised regulations in place to prevent discrimination on the grounds of race or sex but there are no regulations to prevent discrimination on grounds of age; as usual, anything to do with age - even at 50 - receives no consideration whatever.

Society has been allowed to develop so that elder workers and elder folk generally are the last in any queue. Society has been allowed to develop so that if you're doing well you'll do better but if you're having a hard time you'll be sure to suffer more.

The wealthiest people in the country have been allowed a 62% increase in their earnings in the past fifteen years while the poorest have had no increase at all in the same period.

In addition to the lack of employment situation facing Over 55s, from the age of 55 you need to be concerned that the two most important aspects of retirement, pensions and an efficient Health Service, will be available to you when you reach pension age.

Judging by the examples of Government incompetence and mismanagement revealed in earlier pages, the future of adequate pensions and a full Health Service is in doubt unless the Over 55s do something about it now.

At the present time pensioners in the U.K. do not enjoy pensions as good as those in other European countries, and medical treatment is being increasingly denied to older people solely on grounds of age in many parts of the country. It is a fact that the pensioners who won the war are 40% worse off than the pensioners who lost the war.

Apart from the age factor, it is no wonder that Government money is squandered in all directions, 'soft touch' welfare taking one sixth of the National Income, plus scandalous waste of resources by the N.H.S. and other departments, when you have a Government of amateurs, compared to the majority of those in charge of really big business.

Compared to big business, the large enterprise of Government can hardly be considered successful, having got itself into the financial mess of having to borrow untold billions constantly simply to balance the books. Mismanagement and incompetence were the reasons for this sad state of affairs and the Departments of Social Security and Health the principal culprits. The Ministers responsible for the financial disasters of these Departments were both under 50 years of age.

The experience gained by age seems to matter when it comes to the control and management of companies for, according to the Institute of Directors, 29% of directors of major U.K. companies, (over £1 billion turnover), are aged 55 to 59 and 33% are over 60. Nearly eight hundred of non-executive chairman of major U.K. companies are over 60, twentynine are over 80 and three are over 90.

Whatever it is that makes us tick at various ages, therefore, it seems that, to be in control of any successful enterprise, particularly a large one, you need to be in the Elderly age group and, in turn, the fact of being in such a position has the effect of keeping you ticking satisfactorily. Financial and business success seems to come with the experience and sure footedness of age.

With age comes the patience and wisdom to listen to other people. As though the financial disasters were not enough, the splendid structure of the National Health Service is being destroyed by ill considered changes that ignore the advice of experts. The Bishop of Birmingham, addressing a congregation of the British Medical Association recently, said that applying a market system to the N.H.S. was wrong. "Priorities and policies come to be determined not on the basis of human need," he said, "but in accordance with accounting policies. Competition introduced into the Health Service was setting doctor against doctor and hospital against hospital. Men and women who have given a lifetime of devoted hospital service, find themselves losing heart." The Bishop's attack on the N.H.S. changes was supported by the B.M.A).

Of course Government have social responsibilities but they still need to make the right financial decisions. And big business can be successful but socially harmful, the Guinness affair being an extreme example. There have probably been many, many takeovers of companies that have benefited nobody but the successful bidder, and left the taxpayer to pick the bill for lost jobs and derelict communities.

But purely in terms of non-physical achievement there are probably more Over 55s than Under. Consider, for example, Churchill and the men who directed the winning of the war. Consider well known Over 70 business tycoons like Hanson and Rowland.

If you are Over 55 you most definitely have something to offer yet, with present Government experience limiting resources, you are not likely to have any opportunities because the Elderly are the last in any queue when money is short. No alternative political party offers business experience or, for that matter, much experience of anything.

If you are Over 55 you should realise that you don't have to hang around hoping for one or the other of the present political parties to do something for you, or create a situation where the Elderly will have a better deal.

If you are Over 55 you should be fired up by the realisation that the voting strength of the Over 55s, (14,667,949), is greater than any of the other political parties and that you can have a political party of your own, say the ELDER PARTY, (see the comparitive figures in Chapter Ten.

In claiming that the Over 55s have sufficient votes to form an effective political party of their own, it could happen that there would be many EP votes cast but few seats gained, as with the Liberals, in which case this country should have a Proportional Representation voting system. Our present political masters tell us that this system is unsuitable for us in the U.K. for a variety of reasons but we are never told what these reasons are.

You would imagine that other countries would have the same voting system as the U.K. if ours is considered. Taking the following detail from the Eurostat Election Special June 1994, we read that a "uniform electoral system is advocated based on proportional representation - account having to be taken of the particular case of the U.K. which is based on single elections in single seat constituencies."

The electoral system and the most recent results achieved by it are shown in the following tables taken from this Eurostat Election special:-

BELGIUM
Proportional Representation
Christelijke Volkspartij
16.8% of votes produced 39 out of 212 seats
      13 parties represented

DENMARK
Combination of Proportional Representation and majority systems
Socialdemokratiet
37.4% of votes produced 69 out of 179 seats
      8 parties represented

GERMANY
Combined Proportional Representation and majority

system
Christlich Demokratische Union Deutschlands
43.8% of votes produced 319 out of 662 seats
     5 parties represented

GREECE
Proportional Representation
Panellinion Socialistikon Kinema
46.9% of votes produced 170 out of 300 seats
     5 parties represented

SPAIN
Proportional Representation
Partido Socialista Obrerg Espanol
38.6% of votes produced 159 out of 350 seats
11 parties represented

FRANCE
Two round majority voting
Rassemblement pour la Republique
242 seats out of 577
9 parties represented

IRELAND
Proportional representation
Fianna Fail
39.1% of votes produced 68 seats out of 166
7 parties represented

ITALY

Simple majority and Proportional Representation
Progressisti-Federativo
143 seats out of 630
8 parties represented

LUXEMBOURG
Proportional Representation
Parti Chretien Social
32.4% of votes produced 22 seats out of 60
5 parties represented

NETHERLANDS
Proportional Representation
Christen-Democratisch Appel
35.3% of votes produced 54 seats out of 150
9 parties represented

PORTUGAL
Proportional Representation
Partido Social Democrata
50.6% of votes produced 135 seats out of 230
5 parties represented

UNITED KINGDOM
Relative majority in single member constituencies
Conservative
41.9% of votes produced 336 seats out of 651
9 parties represented

Regardless of what it suits our present politicians to

say about PR, there is no doubt that Proportional Representation works well in other European countries, most of whom are doing just as well, if not better than we are. And there is no doubt that, with PR, the Elder Party would be the Number One. We would then decide priorities ourselves, particularly in relation to pensions and the National Health Service.

WHY NOT HAVE
OUR OWN POLITICAL PARTY?

THE ELDER PARTY
(EP)

CHAPTER TEN

The Elderly look to Parliament for their salvation and they usually look in vain, particularly in recent years. During their lives the Elderly have lived through times of strong political allegiance, and have voted, maybe half of their number for Conservative and half for Labour so that their votes have cancelled each other out. In recent years, political allegiance has diminished, with the Elderly resigned to accept that they will be the last in the queue whichever Party is in power.

But now that most Elderly have become disallusioned with political parties of whatever colour, realising the futility of voting for any of the existing political parties, we the Elderly can do much better with our votes. Why not vote for ourselves.

WHY NOT HAVE OUR OWN PARTY?

It is by no means such an impossible dream to have our own Members of Parliament as you might imagine. With our numbers growing all the time we could even form the Government one day. Why should THEY decide our fate when we have the numbers and might have the political clout to decide our own and THEIRS! There are over eleven million of us and this is what polling figures could look like:

Table 1

Conservative	11,057,312
Elder Party	9,202,990
Labour	9,120,943
SDP	4,738,475

These figures are arrived at as follows:-

At the last election, 77.8% of the population entitled to vote, voted as follows:-

Tory	14,048,283
Labour	11,559,735
Liberal	5,999.384

It is not possible to say how many Elderly votes were included in these totals but the Elderly are a conscientious section of the community and may be assumed to have voted at least equal to the national average of 77.8%

The Over-60s totalled 11,829,036, so taking 77.8% of this figure we may reasonably assume that 9,202,990 Elderly voted. Let us assume, also, that the Elderly voted in the same percentages as the majority, for Conservative 32.5%, for Labour 26.5% and for Liberal Democrat 13.7%

Therefore:-

32.5% of 9,202,990 is 2,990,971 from the Conservative vote
26.5% of 9,202,990 is 2,438,792 from the Labour vote
13.7% of 9,202,990 is 1,260,809 from the Lib/Democrat vote

Deducting the above assumed Elderly votes from the actual votes cast for the various political parties, on the assumption that the Elderly would vote for the Elder Party if it was available, we have:-

CONSERVATIVE	Votes cast	14.048,283
	Less Elderly	2,990,971
		11,057,312
LABOUR	Votes cast	11,559,735
	Less Elderly	2,438,792
		9,120,943
SDP	Votes cast	5,999,384
	Less Elderly	1,260,809
		4,738,475

But surely we could get a 100% vote for the ELDER PARTY in which case the EP vote would be 11,829,036, and the figures would be:-

Elder Party	11,829,036
Conservative	11,057,312
Labour	9,120,943
SDP	4,738,475

The EP might also attract Age Group 55-59, since they will want to be sure that a State pension will be available for them when their time comes; and there may also be many 55+ year olds in the never-likely-to find-a-job-again category who would welcome an EP government to look after their interests.

The Age Group 55-59 is made up of Male 1,405,445 and Female 1,433,468, a total of 2,838,913, giving a total Over 55 population figure of 14,667,949.

As before, taking 77% of this figure we arrive at 11,411,664 and

32.5% of 11,411,664 is 3,708,790 from the Conservative vote
26,5% of 11,411,664 is 3,024,090 from the Labour vote
13.7% of 11,411,664 is 1,563,397 from the SDP vote

resulting in

TABLE 2

Elder Party	11,411,664
Conservative	10,239,493
Labour	8,535,645
SDP	4,425,987

How many MPs these figures would produce is anybody's guess, but the Elder Party would be sufficiently well represented to serve the cause of the elderly, and improve the standard of Government.

In three out of the last four elections, not much more than half the total number of eligible voters have bothered to turn out to vote for Conservative and Labour:-

Share of ELECTORATE

	Cons	Labour
1979	33.3%	28.1%
1983	30.8%	20.1%
1987	31.8%	23.2%
1992	32.5%	26.5%

Elderly voters who can't be bothered to vote at the present, and who can blame them, would turn out to vote for their own party, whereas the other parties will always have a percentage of Non-Voters. Indeed, there are many redundant Over 50s who would prefer to place their future, and the future of the country, in the hands of people with real business experience representing the Elder Party, indeed to work for it themselves.

There is no particular problem about forming a Political Party. The SDP was launched on 26 March 1981 and it was not at all certain that it might have a section of voters to whom it could legitimately appeal, not to anything like the extent that an Elder Party would appeal to Elderly voters. The publicity generated by the new SDP ensured initial success but, in the end, their promise failed in the Alliance, a merger with the Liberals that confused the voters.

The 'Gang of Four' believed that a third force could operate in the centre of the political stage, to climb above the Liberal strategy of holding the balance of power. Admittedly the SDP was created to free itself from the intolerant militancy of the Left.

Although the SDP/Liberal Alliance failed to break the two-party mould of British politics, the SDP had twice as many MPs as the Liberals.

The Elderly would not need much persuading to vote for a political party of their very own, say the Elder Party, (**EP**). And whereas the SDP failed to generate any future promise, the future of the Elder Party is favourably influenced, if not guaranteed. Government figures show the number of UK pensioners rising by almost 40% to 14.1 million in 2030 before dropping back to 13.3 million in 2050. At the same time the number of workers will shrink from 34.4 million to 33.6 million in 2030, stabilising thereafter.

When it came to selecting suitable **EP** Members of Parlament throughout the country, for a start there is never any shortage of people wanting to become Members of Parliament, and the Retired have more men and women with senior business experience than all the other parties put together.

There is more to it than suggesting that we put Over 55s/60s in Government to look after the affairs of the country and give the their age group a better deal. The people we would elect would have business, or senior political, experience, which is more than can be said for the average politician. In fact, might it not be the principal reason for our financial ills that we are daft enough to put in charge of vast budgets, people who have no business experience at all. Would ICI or Marks and Spencer or Shell put any of our present politicians, of whatever party, in charge of their financial destiny? Throughout our present political scene, do we not have people of very limited ability in positions of considerable power.

And is not wisdom and understanding supposed to come with age? Middle aged people in charge have yet to learn the folly of their ways.

If it came to the **EP** forming the Government we may not have experience of office but we have as much as the Labour Party and the Liberal Party who have practically none between them. A third of the 1992 Government intake had no business experience of any sort whatever. We would attract to the **EP** members with Government experience if we wanted them. But we would get more wisdom and experience than all the other political parties put together.

The balance of wealth in this country is probably in

the control of the Over 60s so that we would have a better chance of surviving financially than the existing parties, who, we read, are struggling to attract funds.

Imagine the excitement throughout the country setting up our own **EP** organisations. At the moment there are meetings and marches pleading to the existing parties for recognition of the Elderly. The Elderly would come alive with the thrill of having a political party and a cause of our own. The Elderly need a cause to revive drab lives and this would be it, a cause and a chance to decide our own salvation, to change our lives.

ACHIEVEMENTS AND AGE
AND OBJECTIVES

CHAPTER ELEVEN

The greatest threat that this country has ever faced came in 1940. The German Army had conquered Poland, France, Belgium, Holland, Norway and Denmark, flung the British Army out of France at Dunkirk, and threatened to conquer Britain too.

We were on our own but one man did more to save this country, and eventually Europe, than any **other man of any age could have done. Winston Churchill was 66 when he started to lead us then and 72 when he successfully won the war.**

Many of us ex-Servicemen and women saw proof that age is no bar to imaginative, bold and efficient exercise of power. In every theatre of World War Two, Winston Churchill showed himself as an indomitable leader and inspiration. Many of us have personal recollections and mine goes back to December 1941 when, at the age of 67, Winston Churchill came onboard the battleship "DUKE OF YORK" with 66-year old Admiral Sir Dudley Pound, 64-year old Lord Beaverbrook, the Minister of Aircraft Production, and other dignitaries, to sail to America for another meeting with President Roosevelt. The U-Boat threat was at its height, his previous crossing had been in "PRINCE OF WALES", sunk in the China Sea the week before, but nothing deterred Winston.

There are thousands of examples, in all walks of life, of Over-60 achievements As already mentioned, figures kindly supplied by the Institute of Directors show that the directors of major U.K. companies, (over £1 billion turnover), are mostly above the average age of the Government. 29% of directors are aged 55 to 59 and 33% are over 60.

785 of non-executive chairmen of major U.K. companies are over 60.

There are three such directors over age 90 and 29 directors over age 80 of U.K. Stockmarket companies,

A few political examples:-

CLEMENT ATTLEE Prime Minister 62-68
BONAR LAW Prime Minister 64-65
CAMPBELL-BANNERMAN Prime Minister 69-72
NEVILLE CHAMBERLAIN Prime Minister 68-71
WINSTON CHURCHILL Prime Minister 77-81
WILLIAM GLADSTONE Prime Minister 83-84
RAMSAY MACDONALD Prime Minister 63-69

GOLDA MEIR was a sick and tired woman of 71 when she was appointed Prime Minister of Israel but was instantly rejuvenated by the adrenalin of power.
PRESIDENT MITTERAND is 76
Under the leadership of 74-year old President RONALD REAGAN, pride and self respect was restored to America to an extent that would have been considered impossible only ten years before.

There are thousands of competent Over 55s, made redundant by business and society, who would not only jump at the chance of helping to form a local group of EP but who, if it came to it, would do a far better job in government than the present selection. 93% of all present parliamentarians, apparently, have no industrial or commercial experience whatever.

There are thousands of organisations catering for the Elderly, big and small, national and local, where the formation of the EP would provide real interest, even excitement and a challenge.

There are thousands of people with suitable houses countrywide who would welcome the opportunity, and the social side too, of setting up EP local branches.

Famous names would be attracted, (there are more people than you realise who have been passed over, yet in whom the flame of ambition still burns brightly), and they would be voted upon, some favourably, some not. Whether famous or not, there are many retired people of value who would serve.

We need people in power who have the guts to decide priorities, and with tough regard for moral values where relevant, and to ensure that financial provision is available for those priorities - and only then to consider what is available for other causes.

If, as a nation, we go on giving to any cause whether we can afford it or not, we could well end up as a bankrupt country, unable to provide for anybody, the elderly included.

Don't you feel that the whole business of government has got out of hand, that other political parties would only offer more of the same, and that it is time to start anew.

Political parties are supposed to make it clear to voters what principles they stand for, but the major principles expounded by the main parties today seem to be those most likely to secure most votes. There would be no such ambiguity with the EP, however, which would seek to put the Elderly first. In dividing up the National Cake, first to be considered would be an improved pension and then an improvement in the

National Health Service that took special care of the Elderly. To say that the country could not afford this is nonsense; the reason why the country cannot afford it at the moment is because so much money is being spent and wasted in other directions. If the Elderly came first, as they should, there would not be the money available for National Health bureaucracy and other Government waste, nor for giving criminals a comfortable life, nor for making huge awards regardless, nor for all the other idiotic Government bonanzas.

The only reason why the Elderly are deprived at the present time is because they are the last in the queue for everything, and every crackpot scheme is allowed to take preference over the needs of the Elderly. With the potential influence of the ELDER PARTY we would seek to turn this around. The EP political principle would be, "If there's something we can't afford, it won't be the Elderly who go without."

The EP would devise a new set of political objectives and priorities, dividing up the National Cake with the necessary size slices allocated in order of importance, such as PENSIONS to be increased, NATIONAL HEALTH SERVICE to be fully available for the elderly, CRIME, EMPLOYMENT, EDUCATION, ENVIRONMENT and SOCIAL SECURITY to be dealt with by people of wisdom and experience.

If, and when, the ELDER PARTY is formed it will obviously gain votes in areas where the elderly predominate, and it will cause unpredictable changes in most constituencies due to the withdrawal of the elderly votes from their present political allegiance.

There is no doubt that EP would achieve a number of parliamentary representatives from the outset; how many would generate the greatest excitement of a lifetime on election night because there would be no shortage of candidates countrywide. Imagine the thrill, the parties, the adrenalin and the champagne. For a time we would all be fifty years younger.

And once the EP secured a parliamentary foothold it would be on to a long time winning pattern because the numbers of the elderly as a percentage of the population will grow until the year 2020.

If we had the parliamentary numbers we might think of proportional representation and then we would be in power for a long time.

What a cause to get involved in. Come on, believe it is possible. Have a go. Spread the word around. Do something about it.

RECOMMEND THIS BOOK TO YOUR FRIENDS AND TELL THEM ABOUT THE

ELDER PARTY

APPLICATION FORM

NAME ....

ADDRESS ....

....

1. I would like to become a member of the ELDER PARTY as soon as it is officially formed and would agree to pay a nominal joining and badge fee.

2. I would/would not like to take an active role in organising a local branch of the EP.

3. I would/would not be willing to use my premises and telephone as a local branch of the EP.

4. I would/would not be willing to have my name considered as the constituency representative of the EP and I confirm that I am over 55 years of age.
Brief work experience ....

....

Date .... SIGNED ....

An announcement will appear in the national press regarding the address to which forms should be sent.